Midazolam in Pediatric Dentistry

Ashwin Rao · Shweta Tiwari

Midazolam in Pediatric Dentistry

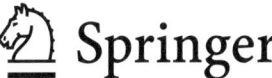

Ashwin Rao
Manipal College of Dental
Sciences Mangalore
Manipal Academy of Higher Education
Manipal, India

Shweta Tiwari
Tiny Teeth-Children
Teens and Special Needs Dentistry
Mangaluru, India

ISBN 978-3-031-45149-2   ISBN 978-3-031-45147-8   (eBook)
https://doi.org/10.1007/978-3-031-45147-8

This Springer imprint is published by the registered company Springer Nature Switzerland AG
The registered company address is: Gewerbestrasse 11, 6330 Cham, Switzerland

Paper in this product is recyclable.

Foreword

In the world of Pediatric Dentistry, ensuring the well-being and comfort of young patients is of paramount importance. This generation of children and their parents walk into our practices with different expectations from Pediatric Dentistry, thus throwing new challenges. As practitioners in this field, we are continually searching for ways to alleviate anxiety, reduce pain, and create positive dental experiences for children. It is with great pleasure that I introduce this comprehensive and insightful book on *Midazolam in Pediatric Dentistry*.

Midazolam, a well-known sedative with good margin of safety, has emerged as a valuable tool in our efforts to make dental visits more pleasant for children. This book, authored by Dr. Ashwin Rao and Dr. Shweta Tiwari, experts in the field, explores the various aspects of minimal and moderate sedation using midazolam in Pediatric Dentistry, from its pharmacological properties to practical clinical applications.

The authors have gone to great lengths to share their expertise, providing a detailed account of the drug's mechanism of action, appropriate dosages, and administration techniques. They also discuss the critical importance of patient selection and evaluation, ensuring that midazolam is used safely and effectively.

As you delve into the pages of this book, a first of its kind and very focused on the topic, you will find not only a wealth of information but also practical insights into case selection where midazolam can make a significant difference in the lives of young dental patients. The book will underscore the genuine impact that this drug can have in Pediatric Dentistry, transforming what might otherwise be a daunting experience into one that is manageable and even pleasant.

In today's world, Pediatric Dentists and their teams strive to provide holistic care that prioritizes the physical and emotional needs of children. Midazolam is a crucial tool in achieving this goal, and this book serves as a valuable guide for those looking to enhance their practices and improve the lives of young patients.

I commend the authors Dr. Ashwin Rao and Dr. Shweta Tiwari for their dedication and expertise in compiling this important resource. It is my hope that this book will not only educate and inform but also inspire those in the field of Pediatric Dentistry to continue pushing the boundaries of what is possible in delivering compassionate and effective care.

Rainbow Children's Hospital Dr. Srinivas Namineni,
Hyderabad, Telangana, India MDS (Pediatric and Preventive Dentistry)

Preface

"*Sedation*" caught our imagination very early in our career in Pediatric Dentistry. We realized that we were duty bound to provide anxious children, with high-quality pain-free treatment even when their age and cognition did not allow them to cooperate for demanding dental procedures. Inhalation sedation with nitrous oxide and oxygen helped us fulfill this objective more often than not. But yet, we learnt in the steep learning curve of procedural sedation that a small group of children cannot comprehend the nasal hood and require other modes to help them through. We worked with various drugs like chloral hydrate, hydroxyzine, midazolam, dexmedetomidine, etc., only to find inconsistent success. Experience gradually taught us that understanding the limitations of these drugs was as important as understanding their indications and advantages. We also learnt that success with sedation should not come at the cost of unintentional deep sedation or the associated risks. As we worked more with midazolam with an understanding of its limitations, this drug started revealing its magic in terms of producing reliable, consistent, and safe anxiolysis, sedation, and amnesia along with a host of other advantages. Proper case selection in conjunction with a good local anesthetic technique proved to be the game changers in this journey.

But, as we shared our successful experiences with this drug at various professional forums, we observed that many of our Pediatric Dentist colleagues were only finding their feet with the use of midazolam. They in their effort to provide the highest quality of dental care to children had various queries on its practical application in practice including case selections, safety, routes of administration, timing of its use, role of behavior guidance, and local anesthesia. We felt a need to bridge this lacunae between theoretical knowledge and the actual effective use of midazolam in clinical Pediatric Dentistry. Therein conceptualized the idea of penning a structured work on the subject eventually leading to the genesis of this textbook. We have nine thoughtfully written chapters and numerous hand drawn figures (Credits: Dr. Shweta Tiwari) in the book. Each chapter has been written with a specific objective to help the reader enhance her/his understanding of "Sedation with Midazolam" and gain confidence in its use.

Here we would like to express our heartfelt gratitude to Dr. Srinivas Namineni, Pediatric Dentist, Rainbow Children's Hospital Hyderabad, a pioneer of dental sedation in India who flagged us off on this journey of sedation in Pediatric Dentistry. He was kind enough to consent writing the foreword for this work. We also remain grateful to the entire Indian Pediatric Dental community for always encouraging us through this exciting undertaking.

We dedicate this book to our entire family whose unconditional love and support gave us the time to focus, deliberate, write and rewrite every chapter leading to the treatise that you are now reading.

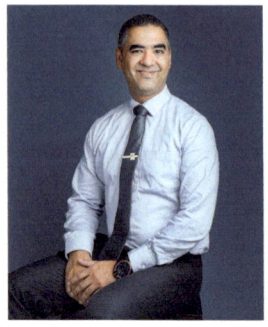

Mangaluru, India   Ashwin Rao

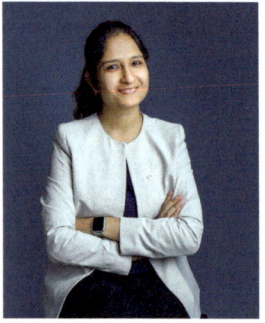

December 2023   Shweta Tiwari

Contents

The Practical Role of Midazolam in Pediatric Dentistry

1.1 Overview

Midazolam has a definite role in the behavior guidance armamentarium of the Pediatric Dentist. But to make its use predictable and consistent requires not only an in-depth understanding of the drug but also an understanding of its limitations. This introductory chapter deals with the need for pharmacological management in children, the roles of midazolam and inhalation sedation, and the unique properties that make midazolam an almost ideal sedative agent in Pediatric Dentistry. This chapter also helps the reader appreciate that midazolam in prescribed doses will lead to minimal/moderate sedation only. Minimal/moderate sedation won't be able to overcome the extreme fear of a combative child. Hence, midazolam on its own will *not* be effective in combative children. It will work best for anxious children in conjunction with non-pharmacological behavior guidance and good local anesthetic techniques, which are ultimately the cornerstones of child management in Pediatric Dentistry.

1.2 Background and Objective

Midazolam is currently the dental sedative of choice in children [1]. But numerous questions accompany its use among clinicians learning the ropes of sedation (Fig. 1.1).

The objective of this introductory chapter will be to address these questions in a nutshell and elaborate upon them in the subsequent chapters.

A. Rao, S. Tiwari, *Midazolam in Pediatric Dentistry*,
https://doi.org/10.1007/978-3-031-45147-8_1

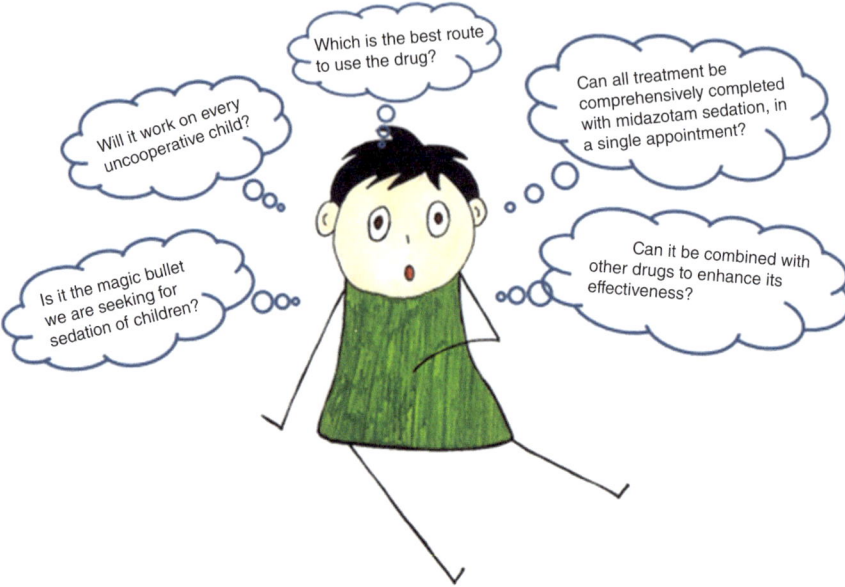

Fig. 1.1 Questions accompanying the use of midazolam in Pediatric Dentistry

1.3　Need for Pharmacological Management in Children

Non-pharmacological behavior guidance with good local anesthetic techniques is still the cornerstone of child management in Pediatric Dentistry. But it cannot be denied that dental treatment even for the most cooperative child can be anxiety provoking and intimidating. This is where pharmacological management steps in, helping anxious children cope up positively with the treatment.

1.4　The Role of Inhalation Sedation and Other Sedative Drugs

Inhalation sedation with nitrous oxide and oxygen along with non-pharmacological behavior guidance and local anesthesia completes the powerful troika of behavior guidance tools capable of managing most apprehensive children. But inhalation sedation requires the child to sportingly wear the nasal hood. Most children do that with good communicative behavior guidance. But age, extreme anxiety, and an inability to comprehend instructions impede many children from doing so. This is where the need for other drugs come into play. Drugs, which will sedate the child predictably for short procedures or facilitate the acceptance of the nasal hood for long procedures. A long list of prospective drug classes become relevant in this space. Benzodiazepines, barbiturates, opioids, antihistamines, and other drugs like ketamine are the frontrunners. Among these, the benzodiazepine class of drugs have currently established themselves as the most effective oral anxiolytic drugs [2].

1.5 The Benzodiazepines

The discovery of chlordiazepoxide, the first drug in the benzodiazepine class, in 1957 by L. H. Sternbach and L. O. Randall represents a milestone in the journey of psychoactive drugs. It leads the way for the synthesis of more than 2000 benzodiazepines ever since [2].

The popularity of benzodiazepines is because of their high therapeutic index. The therapeutic index signifies the relative safety of the drug. It is a comparison of the dosage of the drug that will bring about the desired effect as opposed to the dosage triggering severe side effects [3]. In other words, benzodiazepines have a wide margin of safety. The availability of an antagonist flumazenil also adds to the safety profile of benzodiazepines [4].

1.5.1 Classification of Benzodiazepines and their Clinical Applications

This big family of benzodiazepine drugs are broadly classified as benzodiazepine antianxiety agents and benzodiazepine sedative hypnotic agents [2].

The antianxiety agents are commonly used for pretreatment anxiolysis in adults. They are intended to produce the "minimal" level of sedation usually without impairing the mental alertness, psychomotor performance, and ventilator or cardiovascular performance. Oxazepam and diazepam are popular drugs in this category. Diazepam introduced in 1963 is considered the poster boy of this benzodiazepine subcategory and still continues to be a very popular drug in this category.

The benzodiazepine sedative hypnotic agents manifest sedation, clinically producing a calming effect along with drowsiness and ataxia. Higher doses of this group of drugs produce hypnosis or sleep. Midazolam and triazolam are the popular drugs in this category. Triazolam is commonly prescribed as a sedative/hypnotic in adults, whereas midazolam is currently the dental sedative of choice in children [1].

1.6 Midazolam

Midazolam was first synthesized by Walser and Fryer at Hoffmann-La Roche, Inc., in the United States in the year 1976 [5]. It inherits all the desired pharmacological actions of benzodiazepines including anxiolysis, sedation, hypnosis, anticonvulsant properties, muscle relaxant properties, and the ability to produce anterograde amnesia [6]. In addition, it brings to the table several unique properties of its own. These unique properties have propelled it to be the most extensively used drug for pediatric procedural sedation [7]. More specifically, in Pediatric Dentistry, it is the most commonly used sedative agent with the exception of nitrous oxide and oxygen [8].

1.6.1 Desirable Characteristics of Midazolam

The high water solubility facilitates its intravenous/intramuscular injection without any local irritation [9]. Its water solubility also makes it nonirritant to the mucosa enabling the administration of the injectable solution orally, rectally, or nasally. The injectable solution can be flavored to be administered orally in case commercial oral formulations are not available [10]. This interesting water solubility aspect in the chemistry of midazolam along with its pharmacokinetics and pharmacodynamics has been discussed in detail in Chap. 2.

The rapid absorption, onset of action, and rapid metabolism without the "rebound" effect seen with diazepam makes it an ideal short-acting agent for dental procedures in children. It can be used as a primary anxiolytic and sedative for short procedures or can be safely combined as a premedication prior to inhalation sedation with nitrous oxide and oxygen for long procedures [11]. The short period of clinical action also facilitates a faster discharge, thereby also saving clinical time in a busy practice.

Its availability in various forms as injectable solutions, syrups, tablets, and sprays makes it a versatile drug compatible with multiple routes of drug administration (See Chap. 5). The Pediatric Dentist can choose the most appropriate route depending on the child's behavior.

The other desirable properties of midazolam making it an attractive proposition for Pediatric Dentistry are:

Anxiolysis and Sedation: Most alternatives to midazolam for moderate sedation like meperidine, hydroxyzine, ketamine, or dexmedetomidine have primary clinical indications, which are *not* anxiolysis and sedation. Meperidine, for example, is primarily an analgesic. Sedation is its secondary clinical effect activated at higher doses. The same holds good for hydroxyzine, which is essentially an antihistamine. Ketamine is a general anesthetic drug, and dexmedetomidine is intended as a premedication to facilitate general anesthesia or intravenous cannulation. Midazolam on the other hand is manufactured to be used as an anxiolytic and sedative.

Antianxiety Properties: It is very important to differentiate concepts of anxiolysis, sedation, and hypnosis. Anxiolysis is the anxiety relief or "calming effect" obtained after administration of an anxiolytic medication. Sedation literally translates to drowsiness, whereas hypnosis is natural sleep. Midazolam possesses all the three properties depending on the dosage administered. But it is the anxiolytic property with the minimal/moderate sedation that it causes, which makes it a useful pharmacological agent in Pediatric Dentistry. It calms the anxious child and causes mild drowsiness creating a conducive environment to implement basic behavior guidance techniques.

Anterograde Amnesia: Though anxiolysis and mild sedation continue to be the primary reasons for choosing midazolam, its ability to cause anterograde amnesia is especially useful in children during stressful procedures like local anesthesia. The child may still cry during the local anesthetic administration due to the lack of analgesic properties in midazolam. But, post procedure, the child may not remember how the soft tissues got numb. This property of lack of recall after administration of midazolam is called anterograde amnesia.

Wide Therapeutic Margin: Midazolam has a high safety index. This is because of the wide margin in the dose of midazolam that causes the desired clinical effect to the dose that can cause a complication.

Muscle Relaxant and Anticonvulsant Properties: The muscle relaxant property facilitates a more comfortable mouth opening and insertion of a mouth-restraining device like a molt prop. The anticonvulsant property is an additional bonus in epileptic children or during a seizure episode secondary to a local anesthetic over dosage.

1.6.2   Midazolam: A Minimal and Moderate Sedation Drug

We should be absolutely clear at this point that midazolam, regardless of the route of administration, is a drug safely intended at recommended doses, only for minimal/moderate sedation. The concept of "minimal to moderate" sedation underlines that the drug will only help an anxious child cope up with the stress of dental treatment. Minimal/ moderate sedation drugs will not be able to override the extreme fear of a combative child. They will work best in conjunction with good local anesthetic techniques, which in turn will require the clinician to use the entire gambit of non-pharmacological behavior guidance techniques. The concept of "minimal to moderate" sedation is therefore essentially a triangle where these three components are interrelated (Fig. 1.2).

The above concept is explained in detail in Chap. 6.

A combative child with a true objective fear towards dentistry may try and fight the anxiolytic (calming) effect of midazolam. This may lead to a paradoxical reaction with the child becoming more aggressive and fearful instead of calming down [12]. Hence, minimal/moderate sedation drugs like midazolam should *not* be expected to be effective in combative children or those displaying disruptive behavior. These children are best treated under deep sedation or general anesthesia. The only exception to this rule could be pre-cooperative children (3 years or less) requiring short procedures like extractions.

1.6.3   Deep Sedation with Midazolam

Deep sedation is also possible with midazolam by increasing its dosage or by combining it with other sedatives. But the clinician should be aware that deep sedation or essentially an ultra-light plane of general anesthesia [13] may also bring with it life-threatening complications like desaturations, respiratory depression, or loss of protective reflexes [14]. If the clinician desires deep sedation to treat a combative/

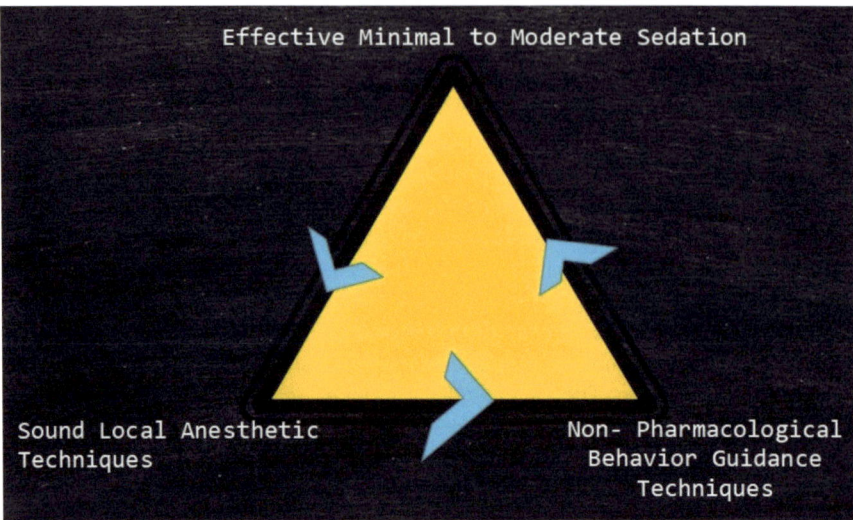

Fig. 1.2 Triangle depicting the importance of sound local anesthetic and non-pharmacological behavior guidance techniques for effective minimal/moderate sedation

disruptive child with objective fears, then there are other suitable drugs like propofol and ketamine which will do the job. These drugs in the experienced hands of an anesthetist will provide deep sedation safely at smaller dosages.

The concepts discussed in the paragraph above are explained elaborately in Chaps. 4 and 8.

We will strive to explain in further chapters the predictable ways to achieve minimal/moderate sedation through midazolam in children. Proper systemic history (Chap. 3), the correct intraoperative protocol (Chap. 7), and meticulous documentation (Chap. 9) are the roadmaps through which midazolam can become a valuable asset in the child management armamentarium of the Pediatric Dentist.

Clinically Relevant Points
1. Midazolam is the most commonly used sedative agent in Pediatric Dentistry with the exception of nitrous oxide and oxygen.
2. The rapid absorption, onset of action, and rapid metabolism without the "rebound" effect seen with diazepam makes midazolam an ideal short-acting agent for dental procedures in children.
3. Midazolam will sedate an anxious child predictably for short procedures or will facilitate the acceptance of the nasal hood for long procedures.
4. Midazolam has a high therapeutic index and hence a wide margin of safety.

5. The water solubility of midazolam makes it nonirritant to the mucosa enabling the administration of the injectable solution orally, rectally, or nasally.

6. Midazolam regardless of the route of administration is a drug safely intended at recommended doses, only for minimal/moderate sedation.

7. Moderate sedation drugs like midazolam should *not* be expected to be effective in combative children or those displaying disruptive behavior.

8. Midazolam has to be used in conjunction with non-pharmacological methods of behavior guidance along with sound local anesthetic techniques.

9. Anxiolysis is the anxiety relief or "calming effect" obtained after administration of an anxiolytic medication. Sedation literally translates to drowsiness, whereas hypnosis is natural sleep. Midazolam possesses all the three properties depending on the dosage administered.

10. Though anxiolysis and mild sedation continue to be the primary reasons for choosing midazolam, its ability to cause anterograde amnesia is especially useful in children during stressful procedures like local anesthesia.

11. A combative child with a true objective fear towards dentistry may try and fight the anxiolytic (calming) effect of midazolam. This may lead to a paradoxical reaction with the child becoming more aggressive and fearful instead of calming down.

12. Deep sedation is also possible with midazolam by increasing its dosage or by combining it with other sedatives. But the clinician should be aware that deep sedation or essentially an ultra-light plane of general anesthesia may also bring with it life-threatening complications like desaturations, respiratory depression, or loss of protective reflexes.

References

1. Wilson S. Minimal and moderate sedation agents. In: Wright GZ, Kupietzky A, editors. Behavior management in dentistry for children. 2nd ed. Wiley Blackwell; 2014. p. 159–75.

2. Malamed SF. Oral sedation. In: Sedation: a guide to patient management. 6th ed. St. Louis, Missouri: Elsevier; 2018. p. 95–119.

3. Trevor A, Katzung B, Masters S, Knuidering-Hall M. Pharmacodynamics. In: Pharmacology examination & board review. 10th ed. New York: McGraw-Hill Medical; 2013. p. 17.

4. Glass PS, Jhaveri RM, Ginsberg B, Ossey K. Evaluation of flumazenil for reversing the effects of midazolam-induced conscious sedation or general anesthesia. South Med J. 1993;86(11):1238–47. https://doi.org/10.1097/00007611-199311000-00011.

5. Kupietzky A, Houpt MI. Midazolam: a review of its use for conscious sedation of children. Pediatr Dent. 1993;15(4):237–41.

6. Gao F, Wu Y. Procedural sedation in pediatric dentistry: a narrative review. Front Med (Lausanne). 2023;10:1,186,823. https://doi.org/10.3389/fmed.2023.1186823.

7. Hinkelbein J, Lamperti M, Akeson J, Santos J, Costa J, De Robertis E, Longrois D, Novak-Jankovic V, Petrini F, Struys MMRF, Veyckemans F, Fuchs-Buder T, Fitzgerald R. European Society of Anaesthesiology and European Board of Anaesthesiology guidelines for procedural sedation and analgesia in adults. Eur J Anaesthesiol. 2018;35(1):6–24. https://doi.org/10.1097/EJA.0000000000000683.
8. Clinical WS, Regimens S. In: Wilson S, editor. Oral sedation for dental procedures in children. Berlin: Springer; 2015. p. 65–90.
9. Kanto JH. Midazolam: the first water-soluble benzodiazepine. Pharmacology, pharmacokinetics and efficacy in insomnia and anesthesia. Pharmacotherapy. 1985;5(3):138–55. https://doi.org/10.1002/j.1875-9114.1985.tb03411.x.
10. Feld LH, Negus JB, White PF. Oral midazolam preanesthetic medication in pediatric outpatients. Anesthesiology. 1990;73(5):831–4. https://doi.org/10.1097/00000542-199011000-00006.
11. Al-Zahrani AM, Wyne AH, Sheta SA. Comparison of oral midazolam with a combination of oral midazolam and nitrous oxide-oxygen inhalation in the effectiveness of dental sedation for young children. J Indian Soc Pedod Prev Dent. 2009;27(1):9–16. https://doi.org/10.4103/0970-4388.50810.
12. Massanari M, Novitsky J, Reinstein LJ. Paradoxical reactions in children associated with midazolam use during endoscopy. Clin Pediatr (Phila). 1997;36(12):681–4. https://doi.org/10.1177/000992289703601202.
13. Ganzberg SI. Deep sedation and GA. In: Wilson S, editor. Oral sedation for dental procedures in children. Berlin: Springer; 2015. p. 157–71.
14. Nathan JE. Retrospective comparisons of the efficacy and safety of variable dosing of midazolam with and without meperidine for management of varying levels of anxiety of pediatric dental patients: 35 years of sedation experience. J Clin Pediatr Dent. 2022;46(2):152–9. https://doi.org/10.17796/1053-4625-46.2.11.

Understanding Midazolam: The Key to Its Safe Clinical Use

2.1 Overview

Understanding midazolam involves understanding its chemistry, pharmacokinetics, and pharmacodynamics. These are the topics where holding a clinician's attention will be challenging. But they are the foundations that will lead to optimal clinical utilization of a drug, and the chapter emphasizes this fact. The water solubility of midazolam, its importance, the reasons for the quick onset of action along with the short duration of clinical action, the safety profile of midazolam related to its pharmacodynamics, understanding properties like amnesia and paradoxical reactions, and utilizing this understanding into clinical advantages are topics dealt within this chapter.

2.2 Background and Objective

"What the mind doesn't understand, it worships or fears"—Alice Walker. Drawing a parallel here to midazolam, a lack of in-depth understanding of the drug will generate irrational fear of its use in Pediatric Dentistry among clinicians. The objective of the chapter will be to provide a detailed understanding of the drug. The chemistry, pharmacokinetics, and pharmacodynamics will be discussed in detail. This will help the clinician better utilize the drug, better comprehend its clinical actions, and better handle complications arising with its clinical use.

2.3 Chemistry

2.3.1 Importance of Understanding the Chemistry of Midazolam

Before this part is perceived as complicated and skipped by the reader, let us get down to the benefits of understanding the drug chemistry. Understanding the chemistry will help you understand why midazolam is water-soluble and the clinical advantages of this property. It will also help the clinician understand the quick onset of clinical action and why the clinical duration of action of the drug is short.

2.3.2   The Basic Chemical Structure of Midazolam

Classically the chemical structure of any benzodiazepine will be a combination of a benzene ring and a diazepine ring [1]. Benzene ring is any compound with six carbon and six hydrogen atoms. Diazepine is any heterocyclic seven-membered compound with two nitrogen atoms (Fig. 2.1).

Heterocyclic compound is a ring with at least two different elements

Side groups are attached to this core structure of benzodiazepines giving way to different benzodiazepine compounds with varying pharmacological properties [2, 3]. Midazolam uniquely has an imidazole ring attached to the diazepine ring. Hence, it is also called as an imidazobenzodiazepine [4]. Imidazole is an organic compound with the formula C3N2H4 [5]. The importance of the imidazole ring is explained in Sect. 2.3.3.

Midazolam is a 1,4-benzodiazepine derivative [6]. This means the chemical structure of midazolam has nitrogen at the first and fourth interface. The chemical structure of midazolam is depicted in Fig. 2.2.

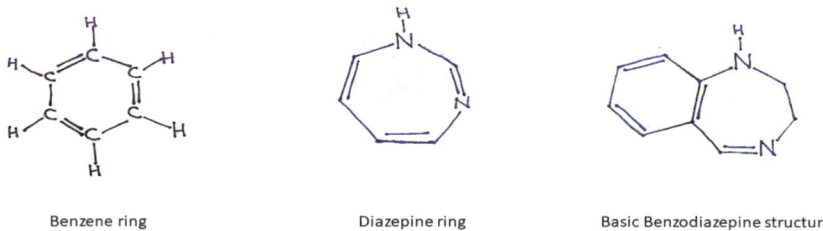

Benzene ring   Diazepine ring   Basic Benzodiazepine structure

Fig. 2.1   The chemical structure of a benzodiazepine

Fig. 2.2   The chemical structure of midazolam

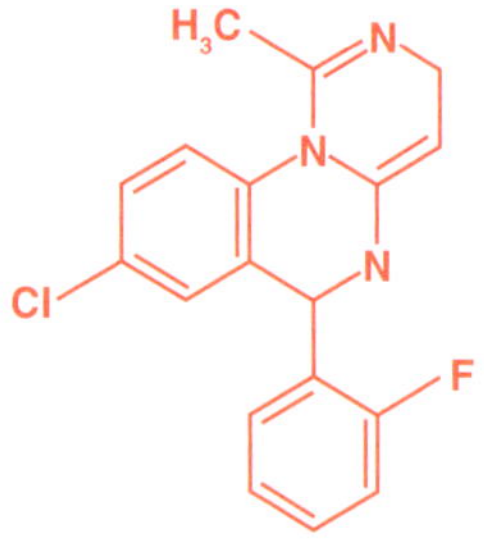

2.3.3   Water Solubility of Midazolam Related to its Chemical Structure

The imidazole ring is responsible for the water solubility of midazolam. The clinical significance of the "water solubility" property is explained in the next subsection. The imidazole ring is a base, thus allowing the midazolam solution to react with acids like hydrochloric acids. This is important because the commercial solution of midazolam hydrochloride (Fig. 2.3) should have an acidic pH of 3–3.6. At this acidic pH, midazolam has about 25% open-ring configuration, which makes it water-soluble [4, 7].

Fig. 2.3 Ampule of midazolam hydrochloride

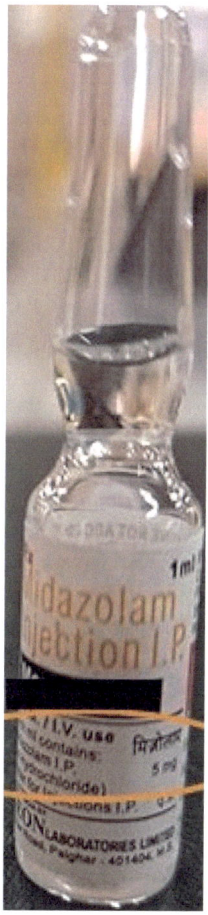

2.3.4   The Clinical Advantages of the Water Solubility of Midazolam

The water solubility of the drug is why midazolam stands apart from other benzodiazepines like diazepam. Diazepam is a very good drug with many desirable clinical properties. But it is not water-soluble. This compels the diazepam injection solution to be mixed with a solubilizing solution like propylene glycol, which in turn is responsible for inflammatory complications like phlebitis [6].

The water solubility of midazolam makes it nonirritant to the veins, skin, or mucosa during parenteral administration. The water solubility is especially a boon for Pediatric Dentistry enabling the multi-route administration of the undiluted injectable solution orally (*squirt method*), rectally, or nasally. Please refer to Chap. 5 for details.

2.3.5   The Chemical Structure of Midazolam Influencing its Quick Onset and Short Duration of Clinical Action

Now here comes the even more fascinating part. As soon as midazolam is administered into the body, at the physiologic pH of 7.4, the rings close making it highly lipophilic [8]. The lipophilic property helps it to cross the blood–brain barrier enabling its quick onset of action.

Its unique chemical structure is also responsible for the quick metabolism and thereby the consequent short duration of action. The methyl (CH_3) group in position 1 of the imidazole ring ($C_3N_2H_4$) is rapidly oxidized by the liver enzymes [4, 7]. Hence, the chemical structure and the pharmacokinetics explained in the following paragraphs are responsible for the short duration of clinical action of midazolam.

The quick onset of action followed by the quick metabolism makes it ideal and safe for short dental procedures in children [9]. It also enables a quick recovery and an early discharge.

2.4   Pharmacokinetics

Pharmacokinetics put simply is "What the body does to the drug." It deals with how the body absorbs the drug and distributes it to the site of action and finally how it metabolizes and excretes the drug. The pharmacokinetics of a drug along with its chemical structure, determine the speed of onset and duration of clinical action.

2.4.1   Lipophilicity of Midazolam

Drugs once administered must cross several biologic membranes. For example, if a drug is administered orally, it must cross a membrane in the gastrointestinal tract to enter the vascular system. This is called drug absorption. The drug is then carried by the vascular system to its site of action. Here again the drug has to cross the vascular membrane to move from the vascular system to its site of action. This is called drug distribution. Crossing of membranes will also be further involved in the liver and the kidney during the processes of metabolism and excretion.

Biologic membranes basically are layers of tightly adhering individual cells. Generally, drugs cross biologic membranes by moving across membranes or moving through spaces between cells, which form the membrane. Since the biologic membranes are composed primarily of lipids, the lipophilic drugs are able to cross these membranes easily [10]. The good news as we already learnt is that midazolam is a highly lipophilic drug inside the human body and so is effortlessly able to cross biologic membranes.

2.4.2 Midazolam's Quick Onset of Clinical Action

The rate of onset of action of the drug is determined by *"How quickly the drug is absorbed and distributed?"* *"The movement of a drug from its site of administration to the systemic circulation"* is defined as absorption of the drug. *"The movement of the drug from the systemic circulation to the site of action"* is defined as distribution [10].

The rate of drug absorption will vary depending on the route of drug administration whether oral, intravenous, intramuscular, or intranasal. The absorption pattern of midazolam associated with specific administration routes like intravenous and oral will be addressed in those particular chapters. What is more important to understand now is the concept of drug distribution.

As mentioned above, drugs exit the capillary system easily by moving across membranes or moving through spaces between cells, which form the biologic membrane. This is where the biologic membrane called the "blood–brain barrier" is different. They are a set of unique capillaries where the cells forming the capillary membrane have tight junctions between them. So, there are no spaces between cells to enable drug movement. So, only drugs that are lipophilic can cross the blood–brain barrier [8]. Midazolam is rapidly distributed and easily crosses the blood–brain barrier owing to its lipophilicity. This explains its rapid onset of action. But its lipophilicity should also raise a red flag when sedating obese children. Obese children may have an additional drug distribution into peripheral adipose tissues, thereby increasing the drug dosage required to achieve a desired target concentration [11].

Once at the site of action, midazolam exerts its action by binding to receptors on the external surface of the central nervous system cells. The degree of binding to the receptor determines the duration of action of the drug. This will be dealt further down in pharmacodynamics. Right now, let us go further into pharmacokinetics by understanding metabolism and excretion.

2.4.3   Understanding Basics of Drug Metabolism

"*The enzymatic alteration of the drug structure*" is termed metabolism. It is also called as biotransformation. The general purpose of metabolism of a drug is to break it down to simpler molecules to enable the body to easily excrete it. It also converts the active drug into inactive forms [10].

Thus, metabolism converts lipid-soluble drugs into water-soluble inactive forms enabling the kidney to excrete the drug. It mostly takes place in the liver. Most drug metabolism in the liver is done by the hepatic microsomal enzymatic system. Cytochrome P450 is a very important part of this enzymatic system, which is responsible for the metabolism of midazolam [10].

2.4.4   The Short Duration of Clinical Action of Midazolam

In addition to the degree of receptor binding that determines duration of drug action, another factor influencing duration of action is the rate at which the drug is carried from the central to the peripheral system. Since midazolam primarily acts on the central nervous system where the blood flow is high, it is rapidly transported to the liver where it is broken down by the cytochrome P450 enzyme system into mainly α-hydroxy-midazolam. This by-product is active. It is also lipid-soluble and hence cannot be eliminated by the kidney that needs by-products that are understandably water-soluble. Hence, this by-product is conjugated further with glucuronic acid in the liver to convert it into an inactive water-soluble by-product *α-hydroxy-midazolam* glucuronide, which can easily be eliminated in urine [12].

It is also relevant to note that the hepatic blood supply increases by 40–60% in the supine position [13]. Since most of the dental procedures under sedation will be done in a supine position, the plasma clearance of midazolam by the liver may also potentially increase during dental procedures. This may also clinically translate to decreasing the duration of midazolam action.

The short duration of action is also another advantage of midazolam over diazepam making it ideal and safe for short dental procedures in children.

2.4.5   Other Clinically Relevant Information Related to Midazolam Metabolism in the Liver

Understanding the major role of the liver in midazolam metabolism may become important if the clinical situation demands its administration in infants. The clinician should remember that the hepatic system in infants is not sufficiently matured till about a year after birth. So, special precautions must be exercised during the drug dosing of midazolam in this age group to prevent drug toxicity. But, when necessary, it is not contraindicated in infants [14]. Practically though, in Pediatric

Dentistry, there may not be indications for the administration of midazolam in this age group.

Drugs like cimetidine, ranitidine, omeprazole, and macrolide antibiotics like erythromycin may prolong the duration of midazolam action by inhibiting the action of the cytochrome P450 enzyme system. Rifampicin will reduce the time of action of midazolam by enhancing the action of the cytochrome P450 enzyme system [15]. But, practically, these drugs are rarely used in children, and hence, these factors are unlikely to come into play in pediatric dental practice. But antiepileptic drugs like phenytoin and carbamazepine are commonly used in children. These drugs are known to induce the cytochrome P450 enzyme system, which metabolizes midazolam. Studies have shown decreased blood levels of oral midazolam and consequently decreased sedative and amnestic effects in patients medicated with phenytoin and carbamazepine [16, 17]. The clinician should be conscious of this fact when administering midazolam to a child on antiepileptic drugs.

2.4.6   Alpha and Beta Half-Life of Midazolam

Half-life is the time taken for the plasma concentration of the drug to be reduced to half its original value. Two half-lives are described for a drug: the alpha half-life and the beta half-life. The process of drug redistribution from the central to the peripheral compartment resulting in the decrease of plasma concentrations is called as the alpha half-life. The alpha half-life determines the clinical duration of action of the drug. It should be remembered that half-life is only the time in which the concentration of the drug in the plasma is reduced by half. The actual clinical duration of action of the drug is calculated by accounting for at least five half-lives. The alpha half-life is approximately 4–18 minutes for midazolam. This translates into clinical duration of action of 45–90 minutes.

The rate at which a drug undergoes metabolism or biotransformation is called as the beta half-life or elimination half-life of the drug [2]. Similar to alpha half-life, a drug does not become inactive past its beta half-life. This is a common misconception, which may lead to a clinician administering more dosages resulting in accumulation of the drug and a subsequent overdosage. Half-life is only the time in which the concentration of the drug in the plasma is reduced by half. It takes at least five elimination half-lives for the drug to be completely removed from the body. Midazolam in children has a quick elimination half-life of 45–60 minutes [18]. But, in general, in adolescents and adults, it is about 1.7–2.4 hours. So midazolam could be completely eliminated from the body, or in other words, the complete recovery time from the effects of midazolam will be in about 11–13 hours. The parent/guardian should therefore be advised to supervise the child at home post discharge from the dental office for this period of time. This should also at least theoretically answer the question of many clinicians wanting to know the interval between two midazolam sedation appointments.

2.4.7   Brief Note on Excretion

Let us conclude pharmacokinetics with a small note on excretion. *"The removal of the drug from the body"* is termed excretion. The kidneys account for majority of the midazolam excretion. An immature renal system as in infants or renal problems like chronic renal failure will therefore increase the duration and intensity of the action of midazolam.

2.5   Pharmacodynamics

The mechanism of action through which drugs exert their pharmacologic effects is called pharmacodynamics. It basically deals with *"What the drug does to the body."*

2.5.1   Difference Between Sedation, Hypnosis, and Anxiolysis

Primarily midazolam is a sedative-hypnotic with anxiolytic properties. It is very important to differentiate the three properties. A sedative drug causes drowsiness, a hypnotic drug promotes sleep, and an anxiolytic drug produces a *"calming effect."*

In addition to its anxiolytic-sedative-hypnotic properties, it also possesses amnestic, muscle relaxant, and anticonvulsive properties. In fact, all benzodiazepines produce these clinical effects in varying intensities through their interaction with the neurotransmitter γ-aminobutyric acid (GABA).

Let's understand the mechanism of action of midazolam in a simplified way by first understanding the neurotransmitter γ-aminobutyric acid (GABA).

2.5.2   GABA

GABA, a neurotransmitter, is a naturally occurring amino acid in the brain, highly concentrated in the limbic and cortex areas of the brain. These amino acids attach to proteins called as GABA receptors. When the GABA neurotransmitter gets attached to the GABA receptor, it causes a general decrease in the activity of the central nervous system. That is why GABA is called as an inhibitory neurotransmitter. In other words, they produce a calming effect and reduce anxiety, stress, fear, and hostile behavior among other actions like seizure prevention.

2.5.3   The GABA Receptors

GABA receptors are proteins that are predominantly present in the central nervous system, though they are also seen in the heart and skeletal muscles. These receptors are present in the synapses of neurons [3, 19] (Fig. 2.4).

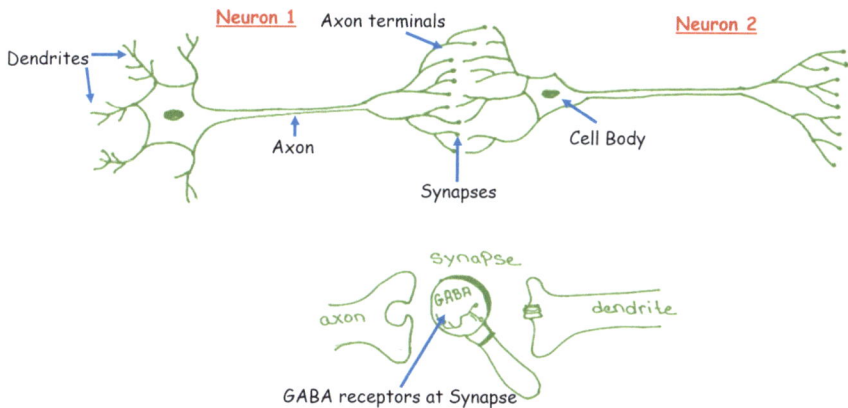

Fig. 2.4 Anatomy of a neuron

There are three kinds of GABA receptors: A, B, and C. Benzodiazepines interact with GABA-A receptors [19].

GABA-A receptors are a protein complex with five subunits (two α, two β, and one γ) arranged in a circle through which runs a channel (Fig. 2.5).

Each of the subunits, i.e., α, β, and γ, is further subdivided into micro-units of proteins. These are designated as $\alpha_{1,2,3,4,5,6}$ $\beta_{1,2,3,4}$ and $\gamma_{1,2,3}$.

Each GABA-A receptor has two GABA binding sites and one benzodiazepine binding site (Fig. 2.6).

The benzodiazepine binding sites are classified into several types (1, 2, 3, etc.) based on the subunit and the micro-unit. For example, benzodiazepine binding site 1 (BZ_1) contains the α_1 subunit and micro-unit. The BZ_2 contains the α_2 units and so on. Each of the benzodiazepine binding sites mediates different pharmacologic actions of midazolam like anxiolysis, sedation-hypnosis, anti-convulsive action, amnesia, muscle relaxation, etc. [19]. This is further explained in Sects. 2.5.5 and 2.5.6.

2.5.4 Reason for the High Therapeutic Index and Safety Profile of Benzodiazepines

When a benzodiazepine binds to its site on the GABA-A receptor, it intensifies the natural inhibitory action of the GABA neurotransmitter on the GABA-A receptor through the following mechanism of action.

When a GABA neurotransmitter binds to its site on the GABA-A receptor, there is a natural influx of chloride ions through the channel in the GABA-A receptor into the neurons causing a hyperpolarization and a subsequent decrease in neuronal activity. A benzodiazepine on binding to its site on the GABA-A receptor, increases the quantity of this influx of chloride ions across the neuronal cell membrane

Fig. 2.5 GABA-A receptor

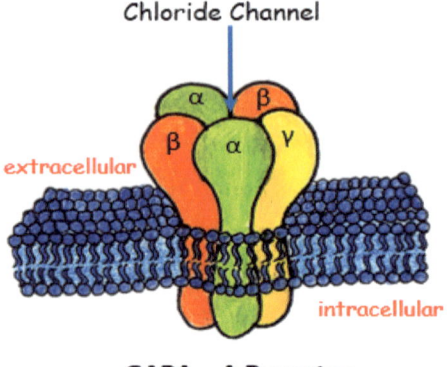

Fig. 2.6 GABA and benzodiazepine binding sites on the GABA-A receptor

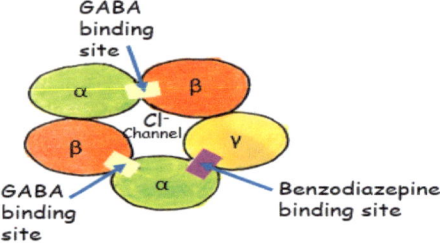

leading to further hyperpolarization and further decrease in neuronal activity and thereby the activity of the central nervous system [3, 19] (Fig. 2.7).

The high therapeutic index and safety record of benzodiazepines are explained by the fact that they only potentiate the effect of the GABA neurotransmitter. They do not, unlike barbiturates, independently open the chloride channel in higher doses leading to severe depression of the central nervous system [3].

2.5.5   Sedative-Hypnotic, Amnestic, and Anticonvulsive Effects of Midazolam

These effects are mediated by the BZ_1 binding sites in the GABA-A receptors. The BZ_1 binding sites are found in the cortex, the cerebellum, and the thalamus areas of the brain that control wakefulness, memory, etc. and are hence responsible for the sedative-hypnotic, amnestic [20], and anticonvulsive effects [21] of benzodiazepines. Midazolam has a strong affinity for these receptors explaining their sedative, amnestic, and anticonvulsive properties.

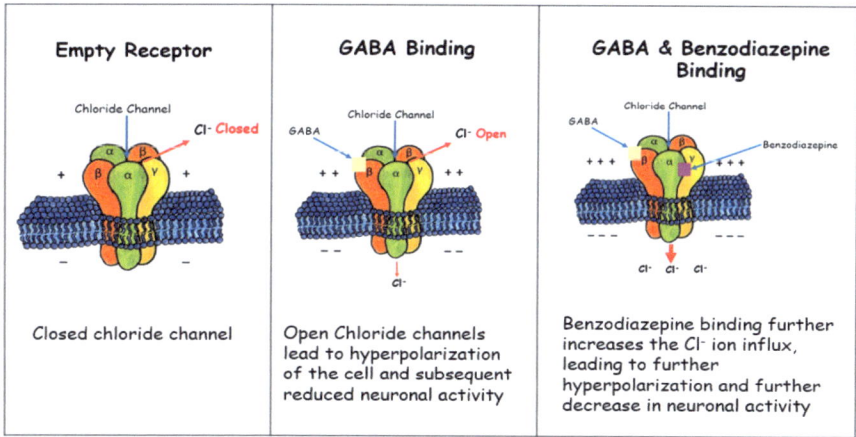

Fig. 2.7 Mechanism of action of benzodiazepine

2.5.6 Anxiolytic and Muscle Relaxant Effects of Midazolam

These effects are mediated by the BZ_2 binding sites in the GABA-A receptors [20].

Let us first discuss the anxiolytic properties, which is our primary focus of interest. The BZ_2 binding sites are found in the limbic system, which is the seat of emotions within the brain. At lower doses, midazolam selectively depresses only the limbic system producing anxiolysis. The reticular activating system and the cortex responsible for sedation and sleep get affected only past the anxiolytic dose of the drug [3]. This selective depressant property as opposed to the generalized depression of the central nervous system is what further enhances the safety profile of midazolam.

The BZ_2 type of GABA-A receptors found in the motor neurons and the spinal cord is responsible for the muscle relaxant actions of midazolam [20, 21].

2.5.7 The Low Incidence of Benzodiazepine-Associated Respiratory Depression

A couple of factors helping the high therapeutic index and safety record of benzodiazepines have already been explained above. They are the inability of benzodiazepines to independently open the chloride channels of the GABA receptors unlike barbiturates and the selective depression of the limbic system by midazolam in particular. In addition, a comforting fact is also that the density of GABA receptors is low in the brain stem where the respiratory center is located [22]. This may explain the low incidence of respiratory depression reported in literature. Respiratory depression associated with benzodiazepines in general and midazolam in particular appears dose related, and no significant respiratory complications are expected until dosing regimens are grossly violated [11].

2.5.8   Anterograde Amnestic Property of Midazolam and its Clinical Relevance

Amnesia is another one of the desirable properties, that midazolam has inherited from benzodiazepines. It causes more consistent amnesia compared to diazepam [23]. It is seen in almost 50–80% of the children receiving midazolam [24]. Also, the degree of amnesia is not route dependent [23]. Though sedation continues to be the primary reason for choosing midazolam, its ability to cause anterograde amnesia is especially useful in children during stressful procedures like local anesthesia. The child may still cry at the local anesthetic administration due to the lack of analgesic properties in midazolam. But, post procedure, the child may not remember how the soft tissues got numb. This property of lack of recall after administration of midazolam is called anterograde amnesia. But midazolam does not cause retrograde amnesia. So, if a difficult venipuncture attempt was done in the child before midazolam was administered, the child will remember the difficult episode.

2.5.9   Paradoxical Reactions

An important aspect of midazolam that the clinician has to understand is the diversified ways in which an adult and a child may react to the drug. Anxious adults enjoy the relaxation and calmness that midazolam or diazepam brings post administration. But a frightened child may not accept the calmness and may try to fight it leading to a more aggressive reaction. This clinical response in a frightened child that is opposite to the desired outcome of the sedative is what is often termed as a *"paradoxical reaction"* [2]. This is the reason midazolam should not be administered to a combative child or a child displaying definitely negative behavior according to the Frankl behavior rating scale. This child (*through good non-pharmacological behavior guidance techniques*) should show improved behavior rating like a Frankl negative, before the administration of midazolam is considered. This will make the anxiolytic and sedative action of midazolam more predictable. Please refer to Chap. 4 for more details.

> **Clinically Relevant Points**
> 1. The water solubility of midazolam makes it nonirritant to the veins, skin, or mucosa during parenteral administration. It also enables the multi-route administration of the injectable solution orally, rectally, or nasally.
> 2. The lipophilic property of midazolam affects its dosing in obese children. This is because distribution into peripheral adipose tissues may take place in addition to the central nervous system distribution. This may necessitate an increase in the drug dosage required to adequately sedate these children.
> 3. The hepatic system in infants is not sufficiently matured till about a year after birth. So, special precautions must be exercised during the drug dosing of midazolam in this age group to prevent drug toxicity.

4. Antiepileptic drugs like phenytoin and carbamazepine are known to induce the cytochrome P450 enzyme system, which metabolizes midazolam. This may result in decreased sedative and amnestic effects of midazolam.

5. The alpha half-life of midazolam is approximately 4–18 minutes, which translates into an approximate clinical duration of action of 25 minutes to an hour.

6. The beta half-life is approximately 2 hours, which approximately works out to 11–13 hours for the drug to be completely eliminated from the body.

7. Midazolam does not independently open the chloride channels of the GABA-A receptor unlike barbiturates. This is one of the reasons for its excellent safety profile.

8. Midazolam selectively depresses only the limbic system producing anxiolysis. This selective depressant property as opposed to the generalized depression of the central nervous system is what further enhances the safety profile of midazolam.

9. The density of GABA receptors being low in the brain stem, where the respiratory center is located, also explains the low incidence of respiratory depression associated with midazolam.

10. Midazolam does not have analgesic properties. But improved pain perception resulting from the anxiolytic and sedative actions and the anterograde amnesia that may follow helps the child cope up with a stressful procedure like local anesthesia.

11. Midazolam should not be administered to a combative or a child displaying definitely negative behavior according to the Frankl behavior rating scale because a "paradoxical reaction" may ensue. The behavior rating of the child should first be improved with traditional behavior guidance techniques before the administration of midazolam is considered to make its anxiolytic and sedative actions more predictable.

References

1. Riss J, Cloyd J, Gates J, Collins S. Benzodiazepines in epilepsy: pharmacology and pharmacokinetics. Acta Neurol Scand. 2008;118(2):69–86. https://doi.org/10.1111/j.1600-0404.2008.01004.x.

2. Batlle E, Lizano E, Vinas M, Pujol MD. Benzodiazepines and new derivatives: description, analysis, and organic synthesis. In: Intechopen. November 5, 2018. https://www.intechopen.com/books/medicinal-chemistry/1-4-benzodiazepines-and-new-derivatives-description-analysis-and-organic-synthesis. Accessed 21 July 2020. Doi: https://doi.org/10.5772/interchopen.79879.

3. Gerecke M. Chemical structure and properties of midazolam compared with other benzodiazepines. Br J Clin Pharmacol. 1983;16 Suppl 1:11S–6S. https://doi.org/10.1111/j.1365-2125.1983.tb02266.x.

4. Pieri L. Preclinical pharmacology of midazolam. Br J Clin Pharmacol. 1983;16 Suppl 1:17S–27S. https://doi.org/10.1111/j.1365-2125.1983.tb02267.x.
5. Imidazole. In: Wikipedia the free encyclopedia. https://en.wikipedia.org/wiki/Imidazole. Accessed 21 July 2020.
6. Pharmacology. In: Malamed SJ, editor. Sedation: a guide to patient management, 6th ed. St. Louis: Mosby Elsevier; 2010, pp. 319–58.
7. Kanto JH. Midazolam: the first water-soluble benzodiazepine. Pharmacology, pharmacokinetics and efficacy in insomnia and anesthesia. Pharmacotherapy. 1985;5(3):138–55. https://doi.org/10.1002/j.1875-9114.1985.tb03411.x.
8. Pieri L, Schaffner R, Scherschlicht R, et al. Pharmacology of midazolam. Arzneimittelforschung. 1981;31(12a):2180–201.
9. Walbergh EJ, Wills RJ, Eckhert J. Plasma concentrations of midazolam in children following intranasal administration. Anesthesiology. 1991;74(2):233–5. https://doi.org/10.1097/00000542-199102000-00007.
10. Pharmacokinetics, pharmacodynamics, and drug interactions. In: Basic medical key https://basicmedicalkey.com/pharmacokinetics-pharmacodynamics-and-drug-interactions/. Accessed 21 July 2020.
11. Reves JG, Fragen RJ, Vinik HR, Greenblatt DJ. Midazolam: pharmacology and uses. Anesthesiology. 1985;62(3):310–24.
12. Midazolam. In: DrugBank. https://www.drugbank.ca/drugs/DB00683. Accessed 21 July 2020.
13. Kanto J, Allonen H. Pharmacokinetics and the sedative effect of midazolam. Int J Clin Pharmacol Ther Toxicol. 1983;21(9):460–3.
14. Pacifici GM. Clinical pharmacology of midazolam in neonates and children: effect of disease-a review. Int J Pediatr. 2014;2014:309342. https://doi.org/10.1155/2014/309342. Epub 2014 Feb 18.
15. Alzahrani AM, Wyne AH. Use of oral midazolam sedation in pediatric dentistry: a review. Pak Oral Dent J. 2012;32(3):444–55.
16. Backman JT, Olkkola KT, Ojala M, Laaksovirta H, Neuvonen PJ. Concentrations and effects of oral midazolam are greatly reduced in patients treated with carbamazepine or phenytoin. Epilepsia. 1996;37(3):253–7. https://doi.org/10.1111/j.1528-1157.1996.tb00021.x.
17. Hayashi T, Higuchi H, Tomoyasu Y, Ishii-Maruhama M, Maeda S, Miyawaki T. Effect of carbamazepine or phenytoin therapy on blood level of intravenously administered midazolam: a prospective cohort study. J Anesth. 2016;30(1):166–9. https://doi.org/10.1007/s00540-015-2063-3.
18. Payne K, Mattheyse FJ, Liebenberg D, Dawes T. The pharmacokinetics of midazolam in paediatric patients. Eur J Clin Pharmacol. 1989;37(3):267–72. https://doi.org/10.1007/BF00679782.
19. Griffin CE 3rd, Kaye AM, Bueno FR, Kaye AD. Benzodiazepine pharmacology and central nervous system-mediated effects. Ochsner J. 2013;13(2):214–23.
20. Kaufmann WA, Humpel C, Alheid GF, Marksteiner J. Compartmentation of alpha 1 and alpha 2 GABA(A) receptor subunits within rat extended amygdala: implications for benzodiazepine action. Brain Res. 2003;964(1):91–9. https://doi.org/10.1016/s0006-8993(02)04082-9.
21. Crestani F, Löw K, Keist R, Mandelli M, Möhler H, Rudolph U. Molecular targets for the myorelaxant action of diazepam. Mol Pharmacol. 2001;59(3):442–5. https://doi.org/10.1124/mol.59.3.442.
22. Study RE, Barker JL. Cellular mechanisms of benzodiazepine action. JAMA. 1982;247(15):2147–51.
23. Kupietzky A, Houpt MI. Midazolam: a review of its use for conscious sedation of children. Pediatr Dent. 1993;15(4):237–41.
24. Payne KA, Coetzee AR, Mattheyse FJ. Midazolam and amnesia in pediatric premedication. Acta Anaesthesiol Belg. 1991;42:101–5.

Pre-operative Assessment: The Key to Safe Sedation Outcomes

3

3.1 Overview

Midazolam is a very safe drug by all counts. A sound knowledge of the child's systemic background will further enhance its safety profile by aiding the clinician select cases confidently or refer the child for further medical evaluation, when in doubt. Either ways, a structured pre-operative assessment will, as the title of the chapter suggests, be the key for safe sedation outcomes. This chapter is intended to systematically structure pre-operative assessment, prior to sedation in the dental OPD. The importance of categorizing the child under the American Society of Anesthesiologists (ASA) classification and the steps to get there is explained. The steps are practical and can be easily accomplished in a dental office. The auscultation process, which is infrequently discussed in a pediatric dental curriculum prior to planning sedation, is also explained and simplified in this chapter.

3.2 Background and Objective

When sedation to accomplish the dental treatment for the child is proposed to the parent, more often than not the parents voice their concern about the safety of the procedure. Here the clinician rightfully reassures the parent regarding the established safety record of minimal/moderate sedation in general. But how does the clinician reassure herself/himself that no unexpected complications will happen during the sedation episode? This is where the clinician has to answer the following important question:

What is the American Society of Anesthesiologists (ASA) classification for this child?

This chapter will elaborate on the process leading to the answer of this question.

© The Author(s), under exclusive license to Springer Nature Switzerland AG 2024
A. Rao, S. Tiwari, *Midazolam in Pediatric Dentistry*,
https://doi.org/10.1007/978-3-031-45147-8_3

ASA I	A normal healthy patient
ASA II	A patient with mild systemic disease (e.g., controlled reactive airway disease which may include a variety of signs and symptoms including coughing, wheezing or asthma)
ASA III	A patient with severe systemic disease (e.g., an actively wheezing child)
ASA IV	A patient with severe systemic disease that is a constant threat to life (e.g., a child diagnosed with status asthmaticus)
ASA V	A moribund patient who is not expected to survive without the operation (e.g., a child diagnosed with a severe cardiomyopathy recommended a heart transplantation)

Fig. 3.1 The American Society of Anesthesiologists (*ASA*) classification

3.3   ASA Classification and its Importance in Sedation

The American Society of Anesthesiologists (*ASA*) classification indicates the systemic status of a patient. It is as follows [1] (Fig. 3.1):

An "E" after the classification would indicate that this is an emergency rather than a scheduled patient.

Only ASA I and ASA II children can be taken up for sedation safely in a dental office [2].

ASA III and ASA IV patients requiring moderate sedation should ideally be treated in a hospital setup or in the dental office under the supervision of an anesthesiologist.

3.4   Steps to Arrive at an ASA Category for the Child

To arrive at an ASA category for the child, seven aspects have to be recorded and analyzed:

1. A structured medical history
2. Evaluation of vital signs
3. Body mass index (BMI) for age percentiles
4. Tonsil size and extraoral anatomic abnormalities
5. Mallampati classification for the child
6. History of upper respiratory tract infection (URTI)
7. Auscultation of the lungs and heart

The reader is referred to Chap. 9 (Annexure 1) for a sample of the pre-operative assessment form.

3.4.1 Structured Medical History

It is an "unglamorous" and often neglected part of the pre-operative assessment. It is often unstructured and ends up as a mere formality with no real information derived from it. To avert this, the parents can be requested to fill a structured medical history form on a printed questionnaire. A short note explaining its importance usually puts the parents at ease, and they sportingly fill out the questionnaire. The clinician can then analyze the questionnaire and discuss further any relevant responses. This way no important information remains unrevealed. The clinician should be alert to any form of acute/chronic pulmonary disease. Midazolam causes clinically insignificant decrease in blood pressure and respiratory rate at usual doses in ASA I and II children. But it can be significant in children with cardiac or pulmonary insufficiency, and their presence should be explored in the systemic history. Any history of hypersensitivity to benzodiazepines should also be noted. Hepatic and kidney diseases are also a concern because of their role in the metabolism of midazolam. Antiepileptic drugs like phenytoin and carbamazepine are known to induce the cytochrome P450 enzyme system, which metabolizes midazolam. This can result in decreased blood levels of midazolam with decreased sedative and amnestic effects. The clinician should be alert to this fact during the pre-operative assessment. Refer to Chap. 2 for more details.

A sample medical questionnaire used in our practice is given in Annexure 1.

3.4.2 Evaluation of Vital Signs

Vital signs evaluation will not only reveal important information but it also is an important form of non-verbal communication. It will help reassure the child and also initiates a good rapport.

A basic physical exam for a child during the "Sedation Fitness Evaluation" will include an assessment of:

- Pulse rhythm, rate, and force
- Respiratory rate and quality of breath sounds
- Oxygen saturation
- Blood pressure (BP)

3.4.2.1 The Pulse Rhythm, Rate, and Force

Place the index and middle fingers between the bone and the tendon over the radial artery near the base of the thumb. Apply gentle pressure till the pulse is felt. A normal pulse rhythm is indicated by pulsations at equal intervals felt at the clinician's finger (Fig. 3.2).

An irregular rhythm could be a cause for concern requiring further exploration by the pediatrician. The pulse rhythm is felt for 30 seconds. If regular, the pulse rate (*heart rate*) is counted for the next 30 seconds and then multiplied by 2 to calculate the heart rate per minute (Fig. 3.3).

Fig. 3.2 Evaluating the pulse

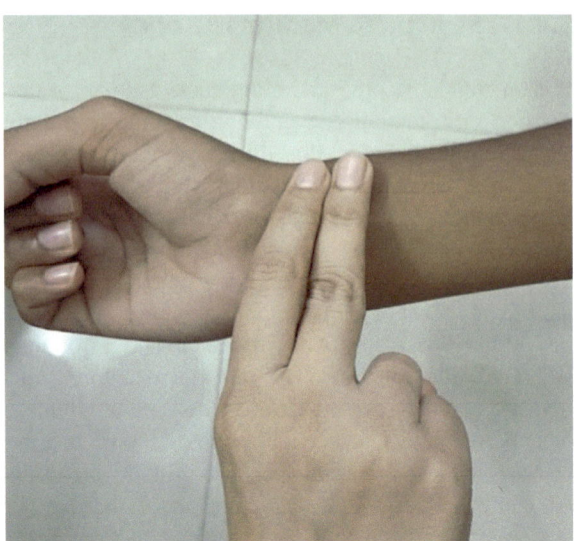

Fig. 3.3 Heart rate at various ages

AGE (In Years)	RATE (Beats/Minute)
Below 1	110-160
2-5	95-140
6-12	80-120
Above 12	60-100

The pulse force is the strength of the pulse felt at the clinician's finger. A weak or a thread pulse may indicate a decreased stroke volume. A strong or bounding pulse indicates an increased stroke volume as during an exercise or in anxiety.

3.4.2.2 The Respiratory Rate and Quality of Breath Sounds

The respiratory rate and quality of breath sounds in a dental office should be heard and analyzed with the stethoscope.

The respiratory sounds are heard best at the precordial notch with the child in the reclined position (Fig. 3.4). The precordial notch is immediately above the manubrium at the junction of the neck and chest. The normal respiratory sounds ensure that the airway is open and clear of debris.

Fig. 3.4 The precordial
notch

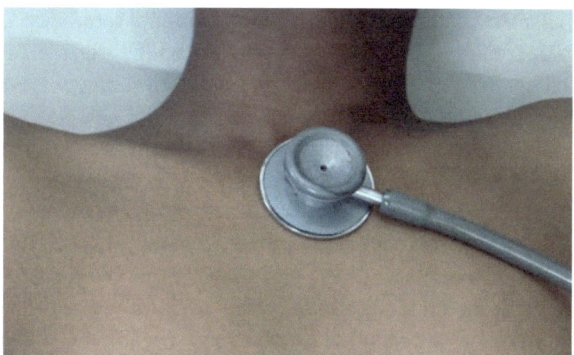

Fig. 3.5 Respiratory rates
at various ages

AGE (In Years)	RATE (Breaths/Minute)
Below 1	30-40
2-5	25-30
6-12	20-25
Above 12	15-20

Breaths are counted for 15 seconds and multiplied by 4 to calculate the rate of breathing. The rate of breathing varies with age (Fig. 3.5). The purpose is to detect tachypnea or bradypnea, which if present warrants a referral to the pediatrician for further evaluation.

> Tachypnea is rapid rate of breathing. Bradypnea is very slow rate of breathing.

Good-quality breath sounds heard as "whooshing" sounds indicate a patent airway with normal unobstructed airflow. Partial airway obstruction is signified through various sounds like snoring, gurgling, wheezing, or crowing.

The auscultation of heart and lung sounds is further discussed in Sect. 3.4.7.

3.4.2.3 Oxygen Saturation

Clinically, the pale color of the mucosa, skin, or blood can potentially indicate desaturation or anemia. But the interpretation of these signs may be inconsistent. A pulse oximeter provides a reliable blood saturation picture. The pulse oximeter probe can be attached on the finger or the big toe of the child. At sea level, the acceptable percentage of oxygen saturation ranges from 95 to 99%. The acceptable range can decrease further above sea levels. Adhesive sensors may be used if the child does not stably retain the clip on sensors.

3.4.2.4 Blood Pressure

The width of the blood pressure cuff selected should be two-thirds the length of the upper arm between the shoulder and the elbow joints. It should fit snug and not too tight on the child's left upper arm. Recording the blood pressure as part of the pre-operative assessment will also expose the child to the experience of the cuff inflating on the arm. This experience should not be initiated first time when the child is under sedation as it may alarm the child. The average blood pressure at various ages is given in Fig. 3.6.

3.4.3 Body Mass Index (BMI)-for-Age Percentiles

Body mass index indicates body fat. A high BMI, for example, may be an indicator of high body fat. In children, BMI varies with age and sex of the child and hence is referred to as BMI-for-age.

BMI-for-age percentiles indicate how the child's weight compares to other children of the same age and sex. For example, a BMI-for-age percentile of 55 means that the child's weight is greater than 55% of other children of the same age and sex. A BMI-for-age percentile less than the fifth percentile is considered underweight, between fifth and 85th percentile is considered healthy weight, 85th to 95th percentile is considered overweight, and 95th percentile and above is considered obesity.

The BMI-for-age percentiles in children can be tentatively calculated by entering the age, sex, height, and weight of a child in any of the several websites for the purpose. The link to the "Centers for Disease Control and Prevention" to calculate the BMI-for-age percentiles is given below:

https://www.cdc.gov/healthyweight/assessing/bmi/index.html [3].

Fig. 3.6 Blood pressure at various ages

AGE (In Years)	BLOOD PRESSURE (Average)
Below 1	110-160
2-5	95-140
6-12	80-120
Above 12	60-100
Adults	120/80

3.4.3.1 Clinical Importance of Body Mass Index (BMI)-for-Age Percentiles for Sedation in Pediatric Dentistry

Now why is BMI-for-age percentiles important from a sedation context? Well, it tells you if the child is obese, overweight, or underweight. Sedation drugs are commonly given based on the child's weight. So the sedative dosage, for example, in an obese child, will be very large compared to most other children of the same age and sex.

In an obese child [2]:

– Fat tissue weighs down on the chest reducing chest wall compliance, thereby increasing airway resistance.
– There may be exaggerated fat tissue deposition in the region of the soft palate and uvula.
– The pharyngeal tissue may be redundant and loose.

These factors may exacerbate the oral soft tissue and the pharyngeal muscle relaxation that occurs during sedation, which may potentially lead to airway obstruction. So in the case of an obese child requiring sedation, she/he still will be classified as an ASA II even if the child is healthy otherwise.

Also, the volume of distribution (Vd) of midazolam is high in obese individuals. If a drug has a propensity to remain in the plasma, then it is said to have a low Vd. If a drug has the propensity to leave the plasma for extravascular binding to fat or other tissues, it is said to have a high Vd. Vd is a useful tool to determine the loading dose of a drug. Drugs with lower Vd can be administered in a lower dosage and vice versa (Fig. 3.7).

So, in general, regardless of whether the child is overweight, underweight, or obese, the sedative drug dosage should be based on the average weight of the child of that age/sex [2]. But considering the high Vd of midazolam, in obese or overweight children, the dosage can be on the higher side of the prescribed range. For example, the prescribed dosage range for oral midazolam is 0.5–0.75 mg/kg body weight. So for obese or overweight children, the higher end of the dosage at 0.75 mg/kg bodyweight may be indicated.

3.4.4 Tonsil Size and Extra-Oral Anatomic Abnormalities

The size of the tonsils relative to the pharyngeal airway is evaluated here. Tonsils occupying more than 50% or more of the oropharyngeal volume may be a cause of airway obstruction during sedation. The Brodsky classification is a useful examination tool here [4] (Fig. 3.8).

It can also be graded as follows [5] (Fig. 3.9):

3.4.4.1 Method of Examination [2]

The child in a semi-reclined position or sitting position, opens the mouth as wide as possible and protrudes the tongue far out enabling the clinician to have a quick peek

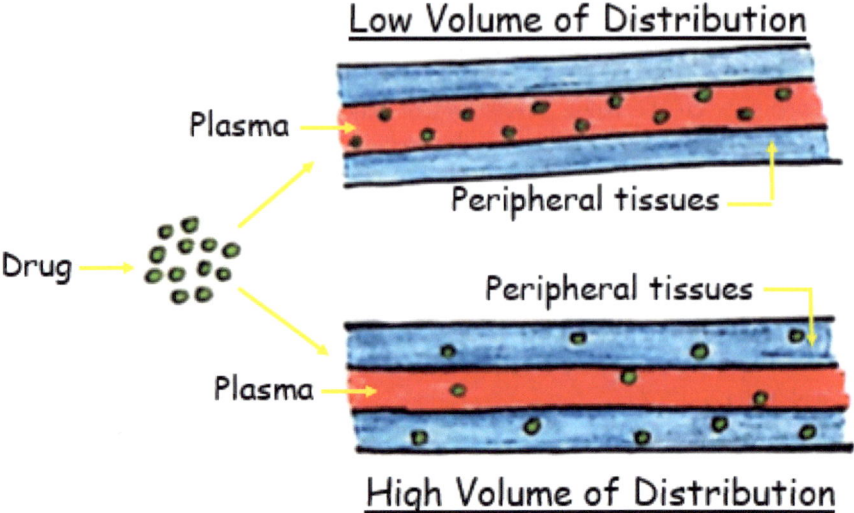

Fig. 3.7 Volume of distribution

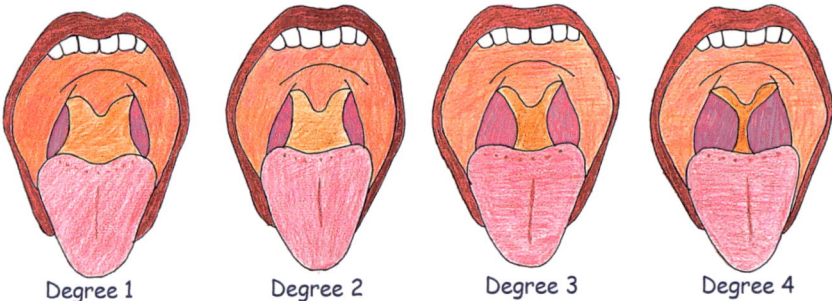

Degree of Tonsils Blockage	Ratio of the Tonsil in the Oropharynx
Degree 1	Tonsil occupies less than 25% of the Oropharynx
Degree 2	Tonsil occupies from 25 to 50% of the Oropharynx
Degree 3	Tonsil occupies from 50 to 75% of the Oropharynx
Degree 4	Tonsil occupies more than 75% of the Oropharynx

Fig. 3.8 The Brodsky scale for tonsil size

Degree of Tonsils Blockage	Ratio of the Tonsil in the Oropharynx
Grade 1	Tonsil within the pillars
Grade 2	Tonsil <50% from midpoint between uvula and pillar
Grade 3	Tonsil >50% crossing midpoint between uvula and pillar
Grade 4	Tonsils meet in midline

Fig. 3.9 Grading of tonsils

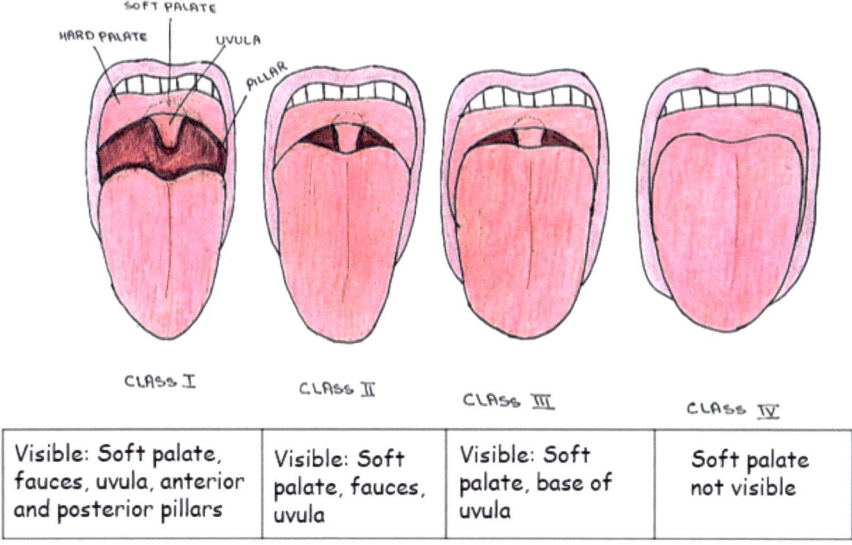

Visible: Soft palate, fauces, uvula, anterior and posterior pillars	Visible: Soft palate, fauces, uvula	Visible: Soft palate, base of uvula	Soft palate not visible

Fig. 3.10 Mallampati classification

at the tonsils. In case the child is not cooperative, the child is restrained in a knee-to-knee position, and the clinician depresses the posterior tongue with the mouth mirror for a quick view of the tonsils.

Severe maxillary hypoplasia or mandibular retrusion, limited mouth opening, severe nasal septum deviations, or obvious nasal turbinates/polyps should also alert the clinician to potential airway complications during the sedation episode.

3.4.5 Mallampati Classification [6, 7]

Mallampati et al. in 1985 proposed a simple examination intended to give an indication to the difficulty of intubation during the pre-anesthetic assessment. As a pre-operative assessment tool for moderate sedation, it can give an indication to the presence of obstructive sleep apnea in the child (Fig. 3.10).

In an upright position, the child is asked to open the mouth wide and extend the tongue. The clinician then visualizes the faucial pillars, the uvula, and the soft palate in that order. The child is graded class I if all the three structures are visible. The child's Mallampati grade increases to IV if none of the three structures are visible increasing the chances of a large tongue occluding the airway during the sedation episode. A grade III or a grade IV along with a history of snoring should raise a red flag to the possibility of the presence of obstructive sleep apnea and should qualify the child to be examined by a sleep physician.

3.4.6　Recent History of Upper Respiratory Tract Infection (URTI) [8]

Check for any signs of active URTI. According to Tait et al., a child with active or recent URTI within 4 weeks is at an increased risk for intraoperative adverse respiratory complications during anesthesia [9]. The results of their study suggested that, though there was no increase in incidence of laryngospasms and bronchospasms, there was a significant increase with respect to saturation readings below 90% and breath holding more than 15 seconds and increased coughing. But they also added that *"with careful management, most of these children can safely undergo elective procedures under anesthesia without increased morbidity."*

The above study in the context of general anesthesia also assessed independent risk factors leading to complications in children with active or recent URTIs. They found that endotracheal intubations in children below 5 years, surgeries involving the airways, copious secretions, children with nasal congestions, history of reactive airway disease, exposure to passive smoking, and history of premature deliveries are associated with more adverse respiratory events. A history of premature delivery has been associated with bronchopulmonary dysplasias and a tendency toward airway reactivity [10, 11]. So are found similar consequences in children exposed to passive smoking [12, 13]. This information should therefore be obtained when recording the medical history. The use of an endotracheal tube has been shown to have an 11-fold increase in the incidence of respiratory complications in children with URTI [14].

3.4.6.1　Moderate Sedation with Midazolam and URTI

In a moderate sedation scenario in the dental office, children with active URTI with active symptoms of sore throat, rhinorrhea, nasal congestion, fever, sneezing, malaise, cough, or rhonchi are anyways easily discounted from elective procedures requiring sedation. It has been shown that the upper respiratory epithelium/mucosa remains sensitized to anesthetic gases or airway manipulation leading to release of factors or activation of receptors, resulting in smooth airway muscle contractions or other respiratory complications for up to 6 weeks post an URTI [15–18].

But the difficult decision is in the case of a child with a history of recent (*severe*) URTI within 4–6 weeks, but is now stable. There is a strong temptation to avoid cancellation of the elective dental treatment under moderate sedation with midazolam in such a scenario. It may be rationalized that moderate sedation involves minimal manipulation of airways, which is considered a major risk factor for respiratory complications. The decision to cancel a sedation appointment at a short notice, also has economic implications both for the practice and for the parents. But it is also a fact that pediatric dental procedures are largely elective not involving an emergency. So, in the above scenario, it is prudent to put child safety over everything else especially considering the limited emergency equipment and expertise available in a stand-alone dental office, in the event of a severe respiratory compromise.

But, finally, it is the clinician who has to make a decision to go ahead with the procedure or cancel it, considering the severity of the acute/recent URTI episode and the urgency of the proposed dental procedure. It is the clinician who has to ultimately weigh the benefits vs the risks before arriving at a decision.

It is the authors' opinion that in a child with a recent history of antibiotics for a URTI, the elective dental treatment under midazolam should be postponed by 4–6 weeks.

3.4.7   Auscultation of the Heart and the Lungs

3.4.7.1 Needs and Challenges of Auscultation in a Pediatric Dental Setup

The clinician aspiring to sedate a child should always do so with a knowledge that the child is not systemically compromised. No stone should be left unturned towards understanding the systemic status of the child. Here is where the knowledge of auscultation is important. The possible presence of respiratory congestion should always be auscultated before a sedation appointment. But, having said that, listening to heart and lung sounds and distinguishing the normal from the abnormal sounds requires a trained ear and mind. This in turn requires auscultation to be done very regularly, gaining in experience and skill to detect subtle differences between normal and abnormal sounds. Practically, this does not happen in a pediatric dental setup. But, in the least, the Pediatric Dentist should understand *normal* heart and lung sounds in the child. In the event of the sounds deviating from the normal, the Pediatric Dentist can then make a meaningful referral requesting the pediatrician/anesthetist to explore further during a thorough systemic examination.

Also, in an ideal scenario, the auscultation requires the child to be disrobed from the chest, which may be unusual in a regular pediatric dental scenario. So, in case disrobing the child is not practical, the auscultation can be carried out factoring in the possible frictional noise from clothing.

3.4.7.2 Understanding the Stethoscope

The stethoscope was invented by a French physician Rene Laennec in 1816 in the form of a long rolled paper tube. He coined the word "stethoscope," which is derived from two Greek words "stethos" (*chest*) and "skopein" (*to view*). He called this method of listening to the chest as "auscultation" derived from the word "auscultare" (*listen*) [19].

The parts of a stethoscope include (Fig. 3.11):

1. Headset, the metal part of the stethoscope consisting of the ear tips and ear tube
2. Tubing
3. Stem, which connects the tubing to the chest piece
4. Chest piece consisting of the diaphragm and the bell

The diaphragm is the larger flat side of the chest piece used with a firm skin contact to amplify high-pitched sounds like the lung sounds and the regular heart sounds. Bell is the cone-shaped side of the chest piece, which amplifies low-pitched sounds like the additional heart sounds. It should be used with a light skin contact.

The following will be a guide to the reader on the auscultation of normal heart and lung sounds. The most important landmark that should be recognized before going further into auscultation is the second intercostal space. This landmark is the one that leads to other auscultatory points of the heart and lungs.

3.4.7.3 Identification of the Second Intercostal Space

The sternum, or the central pillar of the rib cage, resembles a neck tie (Fig. 3.12). The manubrium represents the knot of this neck tie. It has a notch on top called the jugular notch or the suprasternal notch. Manubrium joins the body of the sternum at the sternal angle or the "*angle of Louis*," located at a horizontal bulge 5 cm below the jugular notch [20, 21].

The second rib joins at the sternal angle or the angle of Louis. The second intercostal space will be just below the second pair of ribs on either side of the sternum

Fig. 3.11 Parts of a stethoscope

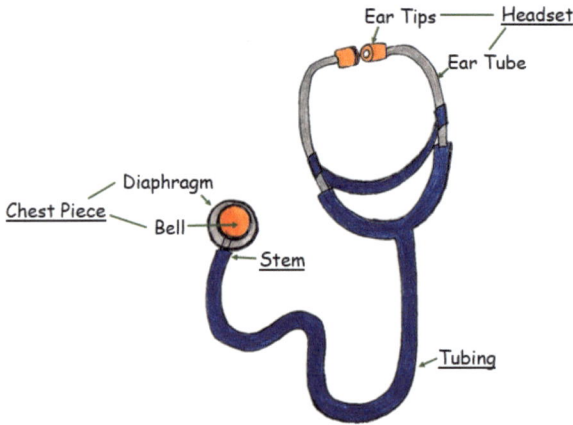

Fig. 3.12 The sternum

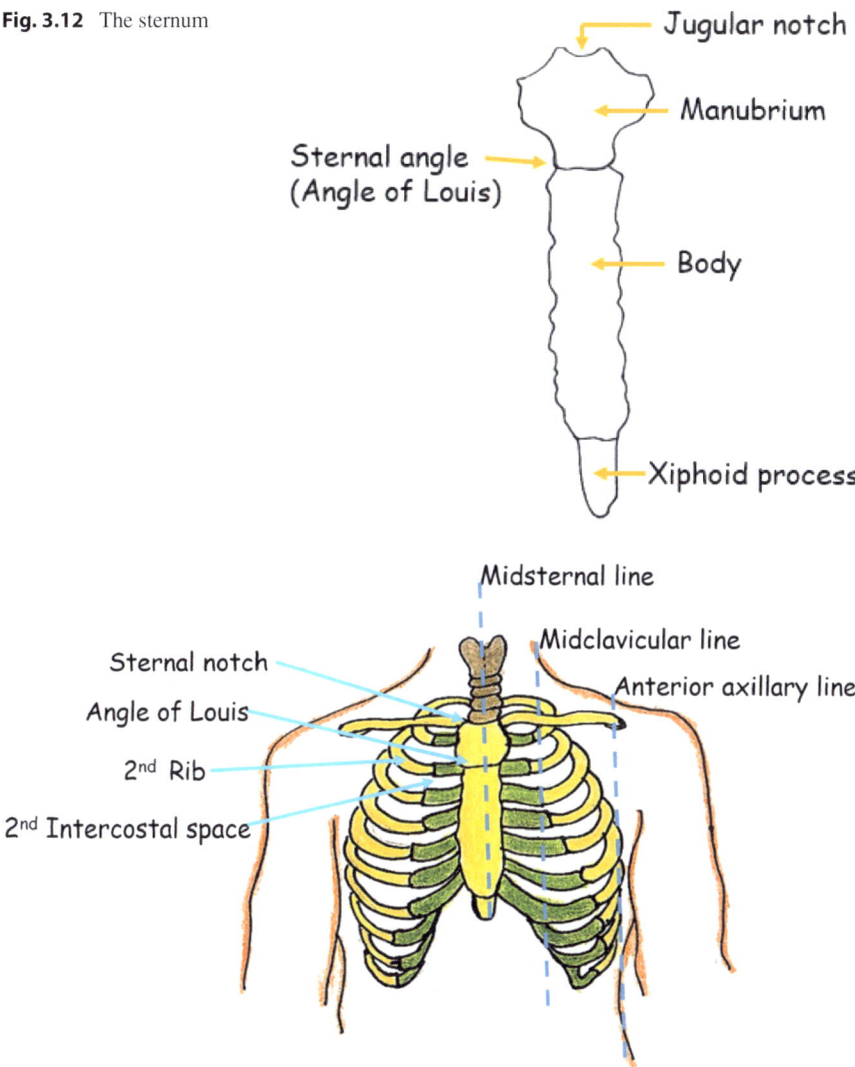

Fig. 3.13 Location of the second intercostal space

(Fig. 3.13). The angle of Louis is also the area where the trachea bifurcates into the left and right main bronchi.

3.4.7.4 Cardiac Auscultation

Basics of Blood Flow Inside the Heart [22]
Let us first brush up on the basics of the blood flow mechanisms inside the heart (Fig. 3.14). Deoxygenated blood from the body flows into the right atrium through

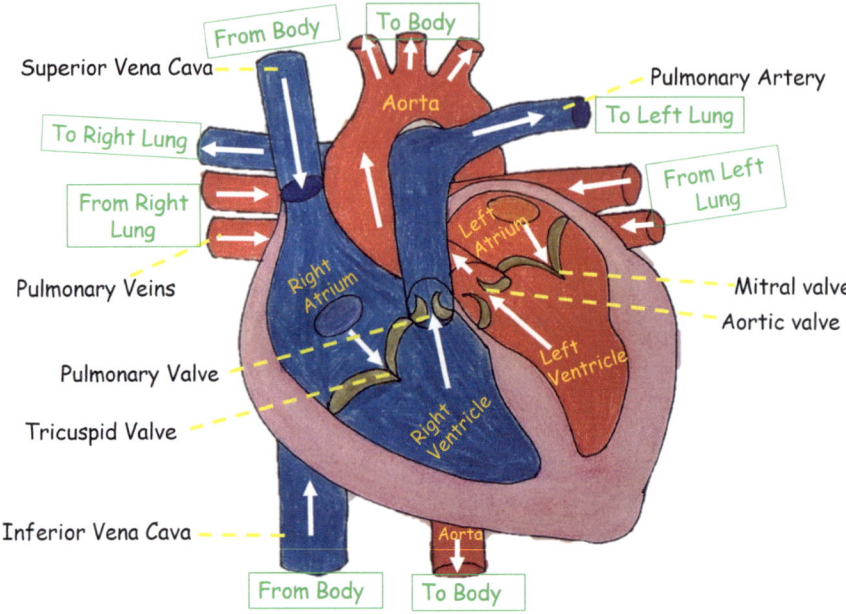

Fig. 3.14 Blood circulation inside the human heart

the superior and inferior vena cava. The tricuspid valve opens and blood then flows through into the right ventricle increasing the right ventricular volume. Simultaneously, the oxygenated blood from the lungs flows into the left atrium through the pulmonary veins. The bicuspid valve (*mitral valve*) opens and blood then flows through into the left ventricle increasing the left ventricular volume. When the right and left ventricular volume reaches their maximum, the pressure closes the tricuspid and the bicuspid valves (*atrioventricular (AV) valves*) leading to the first heart sound S1.

S1 signifies the beginning of the systolic phase. The right ventricular systole causes a lot of pressure on the pulmonary valve, which opens up causing deoxygenated blood to leave the heart through the pulmonary arteries into the lungs. Simultaneously, the left ventricular systole causes a lot of pressure on the aortic valve, which opens up causing oxygenated blood to leave the heart through the aorta into the body. The fall in pressure at the end of the systole causes closure of the pulmonary and the aortic valves (*semilunar valves*) leading to the second heart sound S2.

Sequence and Landmarks to Listening Heart Sounds [22]

The order of listening to valves is simplified by the mnemonic **All Patients Take Medicine** signifying the **A**ortic valve, **P**ulmonary valve, **T**ricuspid valve, and **M**itral valve (Fig. 3.15) [22]. The heart is behind the sternum and ribs. Use the diaphragm of the stethoscope to listen to S1 and S2 with the child lying down or sitting up.

Fig. 3.15 The order of listening to heart valves

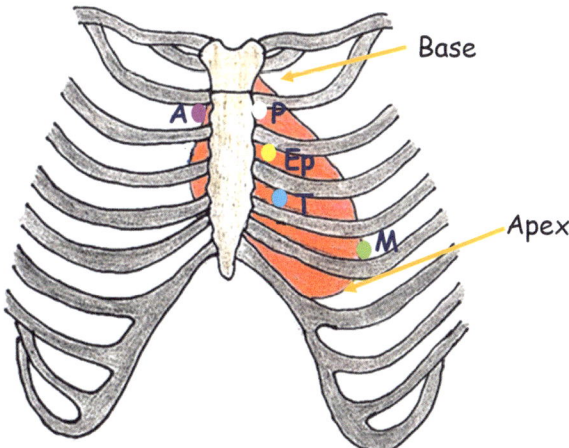

Find the clavicle and find the angle of Louis. Joining the angle of Louis is the second rib. Just below, in the second intercostal space, next to the sternal border on the right side is the base of the heart where you listen to the aortic valve closure signifying S2. It is the only landmark on the right side of the chest for heart sounds.

Now, go across into the left second intercostal space next to the sternal border, to listen to the pulmonic valve closure also signifying S2. The third intercostal space below on the left is the Erb's point (*Ep*) (see Fig. 3.15), midway between the base and the apex of the heart. Now go down to the fourth intercostal space to listen to the tricuspid valve closure (S1). Now move to the midclavicular line in the fifth intercostal space at the apex, to listen to the mitral valve.

Listen to the rhythm and rate of the two heart sounds. To differentiate between S1 and S2, listen in the mitral area where the S1 will be louder than S2. S2 will be louder at the base of the heart. Also, S1 occurs simultaneously with the carotid pulse.

The regular practice of listening to the normal heart sounds will help the clinician begin to identify accessory sounds like the third and the fourth heart sounds (*S3 and S4*), murmurs, split sounds, or regurgitatory sounds. The low-pitched accessory heart sounds are best heard using the bell of the stethoscope. The detection of these accessory sounds will then help the clinician make a meaningful referral to the pediatrician/anesthesiologist for further exploration of these accessory sounds.

3.4.7.5 Pulmonary Auscultation

Broad Outline of Pulmonary Auscultation [23]

Let us first brush up on the basic respiratory system anatomy. The lungs have three lobes on the right and two on the left. The trachea branches off into bronchus and further into bronchi. Bronchi branch further into bronchioles and alveolar sacs where the air exchange occurs (Fig. 3.16).

To examine the respiratory system, have the patient sit up. Ask the patient to inspire and expire deeply and slowly through the mouth. With the diaphragm of the stethoscope, auscultate the anterior and posterior chest walls. Auscultation of the anterior chest will help you listen to the upper lobes and of the posterior chest will help you listen to the lower lobes.

Also note that pulmonary auscultation is done on equivalent positions on both sides of the chest. This is very important to detect any asymmetrical quality of breath sounds or differences in the loudness of the sounds between the two sides. For example, in an obese child, the breath sounds may be quieter or muffled owing to the increased volume of fat tissue covering the lungs. But, as long as there is symmetry in the sounds when both the lungs are auscultated, there may not be cause for worry. If one area of a lung is specifically sounding quieter, that may need to be explored further.

Auscultation of the Anterior Chest Wall (Fig. 3.17a, b)
Start at the apex of the lungs above the clavicle. Listen to the full cycle of inspiration and expiration, and then go to the other side. Next, go to the second and third intercostal space through the landmarks described under cardiac auscultation to listen to the upper lobe of the lung. Compare the other side. Now go to the fourth intercostal space to listen to the right middle lobe and left upper lobe. Now go to the sixth intercostal space (*mid-axillary region or mid-armpit*) to listen to the lower lobes.

Auscultation of the Posterior Chest Wall (Fig. 3.18a, b)
For the posterior chest, the lung is covered by the spine and scapula. So, to get access to the intercostal spaces, ask the patient to cross the arms on to their opposite laps to separate the scapulae (*shoulder blades*). The space between the scapulae and the vertebra affords the best sounds. Also remember here that the right and left lung sides are flipped compared to anterior chest examination.

Listen to the apex right above the shoulder blades on both the sides. Now locate cervical vertebra 7 (C7), which is prominent between the shoulder blades. Auscultate

Fig. 3.16 Basic respiratory system anatomy

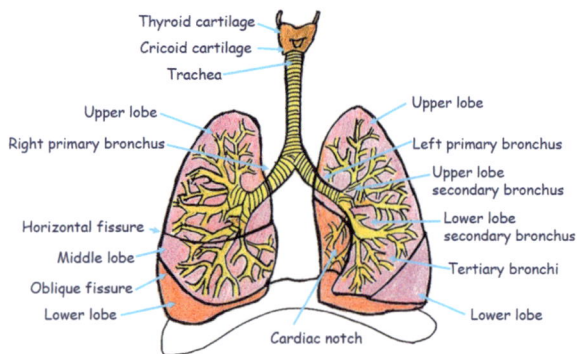

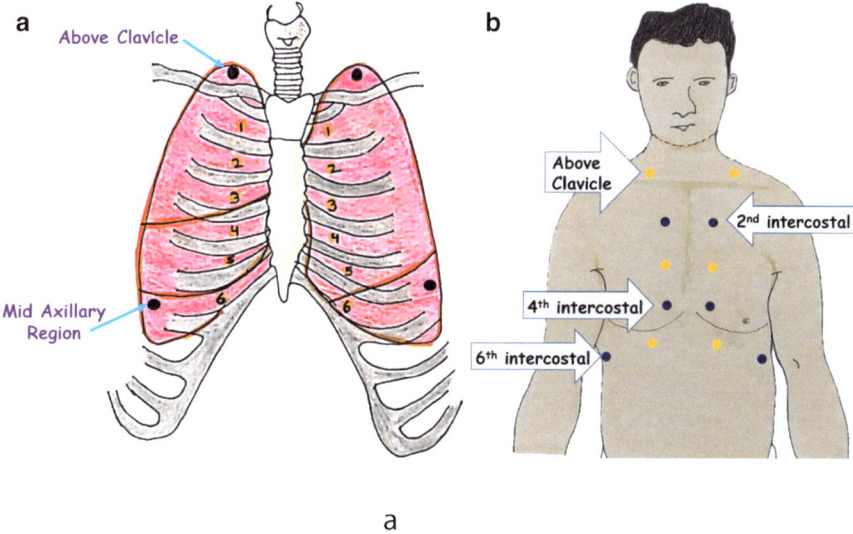

Fig. 3.17 (**a**) The schematic representation of the landmarks for auscultation of the anterior chest wall. (**b**) The clinical landmarks for auscultation of the anterior chest wall

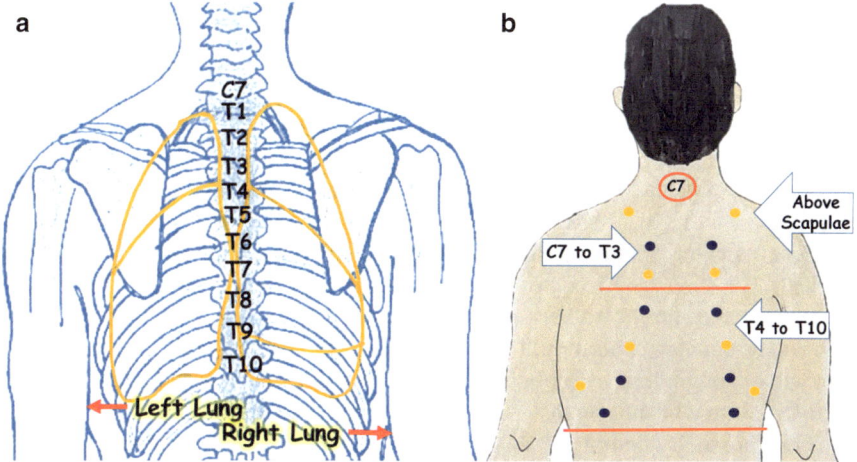

Fig. 3.18 (**a**) The schematic representation of the landmarks for auscultation of the posterior chest wall. (**b**) The clinical landmarks for auscultation of the posterior chest wall

from C7 to T3 (*thoracic vertebra 3 in between the upper part of the shoulder blades*) to listen to the upper lobes and from T3 to T10 to listen to the lower lobes. The vertebral column can be seen in Fig. 3.19.

Normal Breath Sounds

In the above process, listen to a full cycle of inspiration and expiration. Practice listening to the normal breath sounds. Normal breath sounds are of three types: bronchial, bronchovesicular, and vesicular breath sounds.

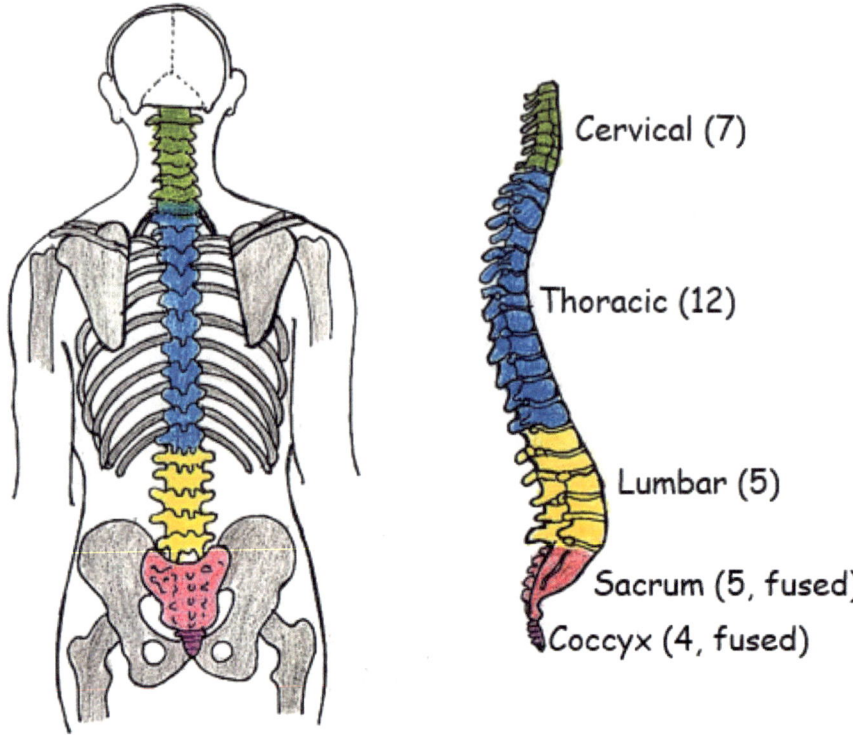

Fig. 3.19 The vertebral column

Bronchial sounds are only heard over the trachea. They are high-pitched. Here, inspiration will be marginally shorter than the duration of expiration. Bronchovesicular sounds are heard anteriorly and posteriorly. They are medium-pitched. They are heard anteriorly over the first and second intercostal spaces. Posteriorly, they are heard between the scapulae in the T3–T4 area. Here, inspiration will be equal to expiration. Third are the vesicular breath sounds. Here, inspiration will be longer than expiration. These sounds are heard throughout the lungs.

In the normal breath sounds, listen to the full cycles of inspiration and expiration, and compare their durations, if inspiration is longer than expiration or vice versa or if they are equal. The breath sounds are area specific and must be considered abnormal if heard over areas where they are not characteristic.

Once you are familiar with the normal breath sounds, then in the course of inspiration and expiration, also listen if there are any adventitious sounds, to their pitch, and whether they are present in inspiration or expiration or both.

Adventitious sounds are the extra sounds that may be heard in addition to the normal breath sounds.

Some of the common adventitious sounds are:

Polyphonic wheeze: A whistling sound heard mostly in expiration. It is high-pitched with many sounds in it. Hence, it is called polyphonic.

Low-pitched monophonic wheeze or rhonchi. Heard mostly in expiration.

Stridor: Are high-pitched musical sounds heard in inspiration because of some obstruction in the airways.

Coarse crackles (rales) mostly heard in inspiration. It is a low-pitched crackling sound.

Fine crackles: Heard during inspiration. It is heard like a fire crackle.

Pleural friction rub: Heard in inspiration and expiration. It is caused by the two layers of the pleura rubbing against each other.

Without going into the diagnosis of these sounds, what is important is to identify these sounds from the normal breath sounds, enabling a meaningful referral of the child to a pediatrician/anesthetist for further exploration. In other words, the Pediatric Dentist must be able to identify anomalies and provide this clinical data to the pediatrician/anesthetist, which may play a crucial role in preventing procedural complications during sedation.

3.4.8 The Sedation Plan Based on the ASA Category

So at the end of exploring these seven areas, the child is classified under an ASA category. If the child is rated ASA I or II, the clinician can go ahead with the planned minimal/moderate sedation by the chairside. If the child is an ASA III or IV category, then the treatment is best accomplished in a hospital setup in the presence of an anesthetist. In case the clinician is unable to decide if the child is an ASA II or III, this warrants further evaluation by a pediatrician/anesthetist.

Clinically Relevant Points
1. Every child intended for sedation in the dental office should be classified under an ASA category.
2. A structured medical history form on a printed questionnaire ensures a systematic approach to collecting initial medical information.
3. Sedation drugs are usually given based on the weight of the child. But the BMI-for-age percentile calculation may sometimes show the child to be overweight, underweight, or obese. In such a case, a sedative drug dosage should be administered based on the average weight of the child of that age/sex.
4. Tonsils occupying more than 50% or more of the oropharyngeal volume may be a cause of airway obstruction during sedation.
5. Mallampati classification gives an indication to the presence of obstructive sleep apnea in a child.

6. In a child with a recent history of antibiotics for a URTI, the elective dental treatment under midazolam sedation should be postponed by 4–6 weeks.
7. The Pediatric Dentist should understand *normal* heart and lung sounds in a child through regular auscultation with a stethoscope. This will enable her/him to identify abnormal sounds when present and make a meaningful referral to the pediatrician/anesthetist to explore further.
8. At the end of the evaluation, the child rated ASA I or II can be taken up for moderate sedation in the dental office. If the child is an ASA III or IV category, then treatment is best accomplished in a hospital setup in the presence of an anesthetist. In case the clinician is unable to decide if the child is an ASA II or III, this warrants further evaluation by a pediatrician/anesthetist.

References

1. Coté CJ, Wilson S. Guidelines for monitoring and management of pediatric patients before, during, and after sedation for diagnostic and therapeutic procedures. Pediatr Dent. 2019;41(4):51E. (Appendix 2).
2. Milnes AR, Wilson S. Preoperative assessment and review of systems. In: Wilson S, editor. Oral sedation for dental procedures in children. Berlin: Springer; 2015. p. 25–37.
3. Body Mass Index (BMI) In: Centers for disease control and prevention. https://www.cdc.gov/healthyweight/assessing/bmi/index.html Accessed 5 Dec 2020.
4. Brodsky L. Modern assessment of tonsils and adenoids. Pediatr Clin N Am. 1989;36(6):1551–69. https://doi.org/10.1016/s0031-3955(16)36806-7.
5. Tonsils and adenoids. In: Ento key. https://entokey.com/tonsils-and-adenoids/#c071_f001. Published 4 July 2016. Accessed 5 Dec 2020.
6. Mallampati SR, Gatt SP, Gugino LD, et al. A clinical sign to predict difficult tracheal intubation: a prospective study. Can Anaesth Soc J. 1985;32(4):429–34. https://doi.org/10.1007/BF03011357.
7. O'Brien SM. Understanding the Mallampati score. In: Clinical advisor. https://www.clinicaladvisor.com/home/the-waiting-room/understanding-the-mallampati-score/. Accessed 8 Aug 2020.
8. Coté CJ. The upper respiratory tract infection (URI) dilemma: fear of a complication or litigation? Anesthesiology. 2001;95(2):283–5. https://doi.org/10.1097/00000542-200108000-00006.
9. Tait AR, Malviya S, Voepel-Lewis T, Munro HM, Seiwert M, Pandit UA. Risk factors for perioperative adverse respiratory events in children with upper respiratory tract infections. Anesthesiology. 2001;95(2):299–306. https://doi.org/10.1097/00000542-200108000-00008.
10. Jacob SV, Coates AL, Lands LC, MacNeish CF, Riley SP, Hornby L, Outerbridge EW, Davis GM, Williams RL. Long-term pulmonary sequelae of severe bronchopulmonary dysplasia. J Pediatr. 1998;133:193–200.
11. Baraldi E, Filippone M, Trevisanuto D, Zanardo V, Zacchello F. Pulmonary function until two years of life in infants with bronchopulmonary dysplasia. Am J Respir Crit Care Med. 1997;155:149–55.
12. Parnis SJ, Barker DS, van der Walt JH. Clinical predictors of anaesthetic complications in children with respiratory tract infections. Paediatr Anaesth. 2001;11:29–40.

13. Mainwaring RD, Capparelli E, Schell K, Acosta M, Nelson JC. Pharmacokinetic evaluation of triiodothyronine supplementation in children after modified Fontan procedure. Circulation. 2000;101:1423–9.
14. Cohen MM, Cameron CB. Should you cancel the operation when a child has an upper respiratory tract infection? Anesth Analg. 1991;72:282–8.
15. Skolnick ET, Vomvolakis MA, Buck KA. A prospective evaluation of children with upper respiratory infections undergoing a standardized anesthetic and the incidence of respiratory events (abstract). Anesthesiology. 1998;89:A1309.
16. Jacoby DB, Hirshman CA. General anesthesia in patients with viral respiratory infections: an unsound sleep? Anesthesiology. 1991;74(6):969–72. https://doi.org/10.1097/00000542-199106000-00001.
17. Little JW, Hall WJ, Douglas RG Jr, Mudholhar GS, Speers DM, Patel K. Airway hyperreactivity and peripheral airway dysfunction in influenza A infection. Am Rev Respir Dis. 1978;118:295–303.
18. Empey DW, Laitenen LA, Jacobs L, Gold WM. Mechanisms of bronchial hyperreactivity in normal subjects after upper respiratory tract infection. Am Rev Respir Dis. 1976;113:131–9.
19. Stethoscope history. In: 3M Littmann stethoscope. https://www.littmann.com/3M/en_US/littmann-stethoscopes/education-center/history/. Accessed 7 Dec 2020.
20. Sternum anatomy review. In: RegisteredNurseRN.com https://www.youtube.com/watch?v=eltLjT8j1r0 Accessed 7 Dec 2020.
21. Anatomic landmarks. In: RnCeus.com http://www.rnceus.com/resp/respthoracic.html. Accessed 7 Dec 2020.
22. Heart sounds explained. In: RegisteredNurseRN.com https://www.registerednursern.com/heart-sounds-explained/. Accessed 7 Dec 2020.
23. Assessing lungs. In: RegisteredNurseRN.com https://www.youtube.com/watch?v=KNrcG077brQ&feature=emb_rel_pause. Accessed 7 Dec 2020.

Basic and Advanced Behavior Guidance Templates Based on the Frankl Behavior Rating Scale

4

4.1 Overview

This chapter provides basic and advanced behavior guidance templates based on the Frankl behavior rating of the child. The traits of each Frankl category are discussed in detail to help the clinician identify and classify children with an accurate behavior rating. The varied clinical presentations of children displaying definitely negative behavior (Frankl behavior rating scale), requiring the need for their further subcategorization to enable a treatment plan, are explained. Accordingly, subcategories for Frankl definitely negative behavior rating are provided to help the clinician build behavior guidance templates based on the traits of each subcategory. The chapter also suggests indications for moderate sedation, deep sedation with an open airway, and general anesthesia under endotracheal intubation. Indications for oral, intranasal, and intramuscular midazolam are discussed. Indications for inhalation sedation and when to combine midazolam with inhalation sedation are also discussed. The chapter reemphasizes that moderate sedation with midazolam is most effective only when combined with sound techniques of communicative behavior guidance and local anesthesia. The chapter ends by outlining a list of practical indications for midazolam in Pediatric Dentistry.

4.2 Background and Objective

Let us assume a situation where a clinician is faced with a child displaying difficult behavior requiring pharmacological management. How does the clinician decide on the intensity of the pharmacological management required? Does the child's behavior warrant moderate sedation only or is the child a candidate for deep sedation or general anesthesia? If moderate sedation is chosen, does the clinician use midazolam, nitrous oxide-oxygen, or a combination of both? The answers to these questions lie in the Frankl behavior rating of the child. The objective of this chapter will be to help the reader accurately classify children, according to the Frankl behavior rating scale. Based on the behavior rating, the chapter guides the clinician devise basic and advanced behavior guidance templates. The chapter also emphasizes that pharmacological behavior guidance with moderate sedation involving midazolam is most effective when combined with sound local anesthetic and communicative behavior guidance techniques. But it should be noted here that the behavior guidance templates suggested for each Frankl category in this chapter do not intend to oversimplify child management. These templates should be used only as a guide and not be considered a "one glove fits all" solution. There may be more clinical presentations of child behavior under each Frankl category. The behavior may also overlap between Frankl categories, and the clinician must sense subtle nuances in behavior and flexibly use the strategies based on the presenting clinical situation.

An important preceding step before the Frankl behavior rating exercise is to thoroughly understand the concepts of moderate sedation, deep sedation, and general anesthesia. The three depths of pharmacological management have been discussed in detail in Chap. 8.

4.3   Frankl Behavioral Rating Scale

This scale was introduced by Frankl et al. in 1962 [1, 2]. It is considered the gold standard among the behavior rating scales because of its clinical simplicity and application. A broad behavior management strategy can be designed based on the Frankl behavioral rating of the child. The four ratings for behavior are as follows (Table 4.1):

Let us now consider each category starting backward from rating 4 with the objective of providing a behavioral guidance template for the clinician.

Table 4.1 Frankl behavioral rating scale

Rating	Categories with description	Wright modification
1	*Definitely negative* Refusal of treatment, crying forcefully, fearfulness, or any other overt evidence of extreme negativism	−−
2	*Negative* Reluctance to accept treatment, uncooperative behavior, some evidence of a negative attitude but not pronounced (i.e., sullen, withdrawn)	−
3	*Positive* Acceptance of treatment, at times cautious, willingness to comply with the dentist, at times with reservation but follows the dentist's directions cooperatively	+
4	*Definitely positive* Good rapport with the dentist, interested in the dental procedures, laughing and enjoying the situation	++

4.4   Traits of the Frankl Behavior Rating Categories and their Suggested Behavior Guidance Templates

4.4.1   Rating 4: Definitely Positive

This child does not present with any behavioral issues in the practice. Two-way communication (see Chap. 6) is easily established, with the child responding pleasantly to the clinician's questions and instructions. The communicative behavior guidance techniques including tell-show-do, ask-tell-ask, enhancing control, positive verbal reinforcement, and use of euphemisms work brilliantly with the child. The clinician though is cautioned against taking the child's good behavior for granted. The clinician should be alert while rendering treatment especially the administration of local anesthesia. A bad experience can easily downgrade the child's behavior on the Frankl scale. Inhalation sedation is strongly recommended during the administration of local anesthesia.

4.4.2   Rating 3: Positive

4.4.2.1 Traits of Frankl Positive Behavior
This child complies with two-way communication and responds to the clinician's questions, *but with caution.* The child is typically anxious or "tense cooperative" as described by Lampshire in 1970 [1].The child will be very alert and will follow the movements of the clinician and the assistants. The clinician must be very conscious of the child's anxiety and proceed carefully.

These children can also present clinically as "timid" children. This category of behavior described by Wright (1975) [3] include typically shy or introvert children. Their behavior stems from an overprotected home environment with little exposure to new situations or people. They may also present as children who follow the clinician's instructions but do not respond to her/his questions. Most often, this is typically a 3-year-old child who is just past the "pre-cooperative" [3] stage. Two-way communication can be established but may require repeated efforts. Here again, the clinician must recognize the Frankl rating trait and proceed carefully. One unpleasant episode may result in sudden loud crying. The behavior rating could quickly change to the Frankl negative or definitely negative.

4.4.2.2 Behavior Guidance Template for Frankl Positive Behavior
The authors routinely prefer one parent of young children, regardless of their Frankl rating, to be in their close proximity and contact on the dental chair at least in the first appointment as shown in Fig. 4.1. The child's feet resting on the parent's lap provides emotional security for the child.

Treatment in children displaying Frankl positive behavior has to be initiated systematically with the establishment of two-way communication. Establishment of two-way communication will pave the way for other communicative behavior guidance techniques, like tell-show-do, to be successfully implemented. It is very

Fig. 4.1 Parental presence in close proximity to the child

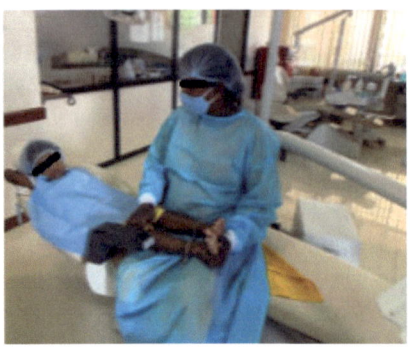

important for the child to get off to a good start. Positive verbal reinforcement by generously praising the child for responding to the clinician helps the child's confidence and self-esteem. This leads the path for a smooth introduction and sporting acceptance of the nasal hood. The acceptance of the nasal hood and the use of inhalation sedation is a big step forward in reducing the stress levels of the child. The clinician should attempt only a short procedure in the first appointment. The appointment should end with the dental team further praising the child's cooperation in the presence of the parents. The child can also be given a gift emphasizing it as a reward for perfectly helping the clinician. Over the next couple of appointments, the complex or lengthy procedures including local anesthesia can be gradually introduced and completed under inhalation sedation.

4.4.3   Rating 2: Negative

4.4.3.1 Traits of Frankl Negative Behavior

Children with this behavior rating are extremely challenging in terms of establishing two-way communication. They *do not* actively resist treatment but will "whine" or "cry" throughout. The treatment happens, but not of the highest quality. Questions by the clinician will not be answered. Instructions will be only partially followed.

The whine or the cry could either be a coping mechanism for anxiety or an attention-seeking behavior by timid or overprotected children, directed towards the parents. It could also be a subjective fear imbibed through parents voicing their fear of dental treatment. The fear could also stem from a previous unpleasant but *not a traumatic* dental treatment experience.

The whining or crying can be very frustrating and irritating for the clinician. A lot of the clinician's patience will be tested and extracted.

Children with attention-deficit/hyperactivity disorder (ADHD) could also present with Frankl negative behavior. These children also *may not* actively resist treatment, but their limited attention span often hinders ideal treatment.

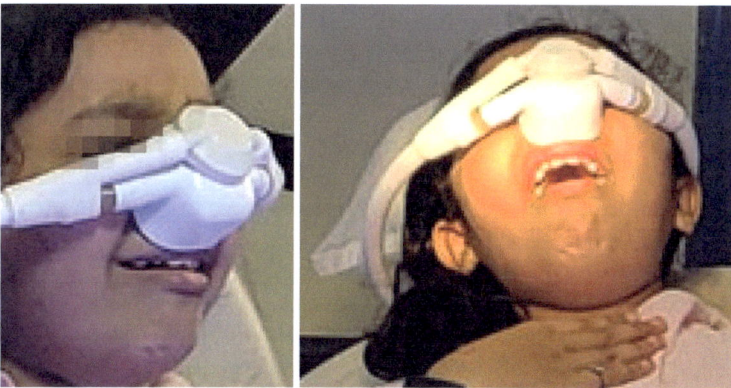

Fig. 4.2 Child displaying Frankl negative behavior wears the nasal hood but does not keep it stable and does not breathe through the nose

4.4.3.2 Behavior Guidance Template for Frankl Negative Behavior

Children displaying Frankl negative behavior accept the nasal hood. But they do not keep it stable nor do they breathe through the nose, thus negating the effect of inhalation sedation (Fig. 4.2). They cry, whine, or move their head continuously.

Premedication with oral midazolam at 0.5–0.75 mg/kg body weight will be very useful in these children. The solution can be extemporaneously prepared by mixing the injectable midazolam with an equal amount of a palatable flavoring agent. (See Chap. 5) Midazolam will calm the child, decrease the anxiety, and generally create an environment where the child will be more receptive to the clinician's communicative efforts. In a nutshell, it will facilitate the establishment of two-way communication. The anxiolysis provided by midazolam will also help the child keep the nasal hood stable. The clinician should not attempt a long or a complicated procedure in this appointment. Instead, it should be primarily a preparatory appointment for subsequent challenging procedures.

Local anesthesia can be introduced when indicated, with a supraperiosteal injection in this appointment. Midazolam facilitates the injection by elevating the pain threshold and decreasing the pain reaction. It changes pain perception through its anxiolytic properties and makes the child indifferent to mild noxious stimuli [4]. Inhalation sedation will produce the analgesia and reinforce the anxiolytic effects of midazolam.

The rubber dam can be applied post-soft tissue anesthesia, and a simple, short restorative procedure with the high-speed handpiece and water spray can be completed in this appointment. At the end of the appointment, the child should be rewarded for her/his exemplary behavior.

The child likely will be in a very positive frame of mind in the next appointment riding on the confidence of the previous appointment. In this appointment, the long (pulp therapy/extractions) or complicated procedures (inferior alveolar nerve block/palatal injections) can be initiated under the midazolam-inhalation sedation combination along with local anesthesia.

If the child's behavior rating improves to Frankl positive in the above appointment, future dental appointments can proceed under only inhalation sedation.

4.4.4 Rating 1: Definitely Negative

4.4.4.1 Subcategorization of Frankl Definitely Negative Behavior

This is the category dreaded by all clinicians. A common characteristic displayed by the children in this category is that they will "actively resist treatment." The challenge to formulating a behavior guidance template is that children displaying Frankl definitely negative behavior present with multiple clinical presentations. They can be defiant, fearful, or hysterical. Frankl definitely negative thus becomes a broad category, which does not provide sufficient clinical information about the specifics of the negative behavior [1]. So, a more practical approach is to break down the category into specific subtypes and propose behavior guidance solutions to each of them. Based on this approach, Frankl definitely negative behavior can be further subdivided as children displaying:

- Defiant, stubborn, or mild fearful behavior likely stemming either from subjective fear or overindulgent parenting
- Pre-cooperative behavior
- Disruptive/uncontrolled/hysterical/combative behavior stemming either from severe objective fear or from specific debilitating conditions like intellectual and developmental disabilities

The above three subcategories can be denoted clinically as **- - 1**, **- - 2**, and **- - 3**, respectively.

4.4.4.2 Frankl Definitely Negative Behavior - - 1

(Defiant, stubborn, or mild fearful behavior likely stemming either from subjective fear or overindulgent parenting)

Traits of Frankl Definitely Negative Behavior - - 1

Children displaying defiant, stubborn, or mild fearful behavior stemming either from subjective fear or overindulgent parenting (- - 1) are *potentially cooperative children* [3], but who *actively resist* the treatment. They may actively resist treatment by attempting to leave the dental chair, loud crying, turning the head away, or closing the mouth with their hands. They must be differentiated from children displaying Frankl negative behavior who may cry but *do not* actively resist treatment. They must also be differentiated from children displaying Frankl definitely negative behavior who show disruptive/uncontrolled/hysterical/combative behavior stemming from a previous traumatic dental treatment experience (- - 3) with a severe fear towards dentistry. The - - 1 subcategory of children displaying Frankl definitely negative behavior may have had a previous unpleasant but *not* a traumatic dental experience. The "defiant" "stubborn" or "mild fearful" behavior could also be a manifestation of fear transferred by their parents or peers narrating their bad dental experience. The "defiant" or "stubborn" behavior may also stem from inadequate disciplining by the parents with insufficient strict guidelines limiting inappropriate behavior at home. They are used to their way at home and hence behave similarly in the dental office. These children will actively resist wearing the nasal hood, thus removing inhalation sedation out of the equation as a behavior guidance tool.

Behavior Guidance Template for Frankl Definitely Negative Behavior - - 1

Voice Modulation

Voice modulation can be an effective tool in these children because the underlying behavior manifestation *does not* stem from a true or severe fear towards dentistry. The purpose is to gain their attention allowing the clinician to communicate with the child. But it has to be done with the parents' unflinching support and consent. The parents have to be assured that voice modulation is a scientific technique where the aggressive posturing by the clinician is only a pretense to open two-way communication channels with the child. Parents usually provide this consent when they are very familiar with the clinician and confident of her/his skills. The clinician may have treated other children in their family, or the parents may have made the appointment on the back of a strong word-by-mouth referral from other parents.

Parents *Not* Consenting to the Voice Modulation Technique

Obtaining consent from parents could also become challenging in some cases. If the consent for voice modulation is reluctantly granted, there is a possibility that the parents at the end of treatment may eventually sympathize with the child and resent the clinician. This is especially true of parents who are hesitant to disciplining the child. They may see voice modulation as the clinician overstepping into their territory and contradicting their style of parenting. The clinician should be smart to grasp the pulse of the situation here and should work towards convincing the parents very tactfully. She/he should show utmost patience with the child impressioning upon the parents the effort and time being spent on their child who is displaying inappropriate behavior. The first appointment can be terminated with the clinician assuring the parents that no treatment will be forced upon the child. But it should be emphasized that although treatment will be carried out with the utmost care, it will be possible only if the parents play a more proactive role in convincing the child to cooperate with the doctor. The alternatives should also be presented, which in this case would be to "defer" the treatment at the risk of the dental disease advancing to a point where general anesthesia with its added expenses may be the only option left. If the parents appreciate the clinician's effort and her/his requests for a more proactive role, the message of the "dental treatment being non-negotiable" may be firmly explained to the child at home. Children instinctively understand parent body language. They understand "when parents mean business" and this may help the child make up her/his mind to comply with the treatment.

In the scenario that consent for voice modulation is not obtained or the parents do not have the will to convince the child, there will be only two realistic ways forward. The treatment will have to be deferred or will have to progress under general anesthesia.

Alternatively, oral midazolam using the squirt method (*0.5–0.75 mg/kg body weight*) or intranasal midazolam (*0.3–0.4 mg/kg body weight*) using the Mucosal Atomization Device (MAD) (See Chap. 5) or rapid induction of inhalation sedation could be attempted in conjunction with protective stabilization after obtaining parent consent. Intranasal dexmedetomidine (*2 mcg/kg body weight*) can also be a very useful alternative to midazolam in older children (weighing more than 25 kgs), considering its availability in 100 mcg/ml ampoules. This leads to very small volumes of the drug that will need to be administered intranasally. But children under the influence of midazolam have shown less combative behavior compared to children sedated with dexmedetomidine [5].

But these modes of treatment should be attempted with the full parent understanding that they are fraught with unpredictability. They may succeed or they may further deteriorate child behavior to - - 3. The objective of sedation here should only be to help the child overcome any irrational fear. If successful, short procedures like an extraction (*local anesthesia should be administered with minimal discomfort*; see Chap. 6), short operative procedures post removal of carious tissue using hand instruments/brief use of a handpiece, application of silver diamine fluoride, or any other procedure which can be completed in a 10–15-minutes window can be attempted.

Long operative procedures under the influence of midazolam are usually unsuccessful in this subcategory (- - 1). This is because moderate sedation drugs like midazolam are indicated for an anxious child who is ready to accept treatment. They help the child cope up with the stress of the dental treatment. But they are not strong enough in prescribed dosages to overcome strong resistance in a child who is *not* ready to accept treatment. Hence, it is unlikely that the - - 1 child will accept the nasal hood, even under the influence of midazolam. Nevertheless, the clinician may attempt the same and if successful, may also attempt to apply the rubber dam post local anesthesia. Occasionally, the security provided by the rubber dam may promote positive behavior and facilitate the long operative procedure [6].

But, in the event of this attempt failing, the clinician should withhold the temptation to overcome the defiant behavior of the child by resorting to a combination of drugs in subsequent appointments. Though the cocktail of sedative drugs may succeed in calming the child, they may also lead the child into deep sedation. Deep sedation in turn may also concurrently bring along complications like desaturations, overdosage, respiratory depressions, and loss of protective reflexes [7].

Pharmacological Management Plan for Frankl Definitely Negative behavior - - 1
Assuming here that the child has been convinced for the treatment through voice modulation or through parent intervention, let us discuss a more practical pharmacological management plan. Even though the child has stepped up to cooperate for the treatment, it is prudent to remember that the child will still be very anxious and the Frankl behavior rating should be considered positive or negative at this stage. The ball is now in the clinician's court. It is now the clinician's job to ensure

that the treatment is carried out comfortably, using sound techniques of communicative behavior guidance, moderate sedation, and local anesthesia. The next appointment is planned accordingly with parent consent.

In this appointment, oral midazolam as a premedication (*extemporaneously prepared by mixing the injectable midazolam with an equal amount of a palatable flavoring agent*) at 0.5–0.75 mg/kg body weight is administered to the child. The purpose is again not to carry out complex treatment. The objective is to use its anxiolytic properties to create an environment where two-way communication can be established and various equipment and instruments are introduced to the child. The nasal hood is introduced using communicative techniques like tell-show-do and euphemisms. Once inhalation sedation takes effect, local anesthetic infiltration for soft tissue anesthesia can be administered, and the rubber dam can be introduced and applied. The appointment ends with a short restorative procedure using the high-speed handpiece under water spray. The child is generously praised and rewarded for the excellent behavior. The following appointments can proceed with the necessary treatments utilizing only inhalation sedation. But challenging treatments like the administration of the inferior alveolar nerve block or a difficult extraction should be scaled only under the midazolam-nitrous oxide-oxygen combination.

4.4.4.3 Frankl Definitely Negative Behavior - - 2
(Pre-cooperative behavior)

Traits of Frankl Definitely Negative Behavior - - 2
They are also described as children lacking cooperative ability. These are the children where communication cannot be established due to their young age (<3 years of age) or specific debilitating or handicapping conditions [1]. But, in the following discussion, we will use the term pre-cooperative to represent only children less than 3 years of age. Management of children displaying hysterical behavior due to specific debilitating conditions like intellectual and developmental disabilities will be addressed in the next section.

Behavior Guidance Template for Frankl Definitely Negative Behavior - - 2
In pre-cooperative children, a two-way communication cannot be established because the children are too young cognitively to comprehend instructions by the clinician. The stage is called pre-cooperative because children outgrow this stage and become cooperative as they become older. Comprehensive treatment in this age group is a major behavioral challenge. But, fortunately, today we have techniques like non-restorative cavity control using silver diamine fluoride (SDF), sealing carious lesions, and Hall crowns, among others [8–10], which help us buy time till the child becomes older and mature. Invasive procedures in this age group are most commonly limited to extraction of maxillary anterior teeth or first primary molars. These short procedures can be predictably accomplished using oral (*0.5–0.75 mg/kg body weight*) or intranasal (*0.3–0.4 mg/kg body weight*) midazolam. Oral midazolam in this case should be administered using the squirt method because the child may likely expectorate the medicine (See Chap. 5). Midazolam effectively

provides a short sedation window of 15 to 20 minutes in this age group, allowing the administration of local anesthesia for extraction or for completion of simple procedures like SDF application, sealing carious lesions, or cementing a Hall crown. The child can be placed on the parent's chest with the head lying over the shoulder, during treatment. This position also helps provide gentle restraint, along with emotional security for the pre-cooperative child (Fig. 4.3).

In some instances, the child may be partially sedated and may continue to resist treatment. The clinician should withhold the temptation to administer the second dose because the effect may be additive leading to deep sedation. The clinician in this case can still go ahead with the planned treatment under parental protective stabilization because of the anterograde amnesia provided by midazolam. Anterograde amnesia is seen in almost 50–80% of the children receiving midazolam, and the degree of amnesia is not route dependent [11, 12]. The child may still cry during the local anesthetic administration due to the lack of

Fig. 4.3 Parent on the dental chair with the child's head on the parent's shoulder

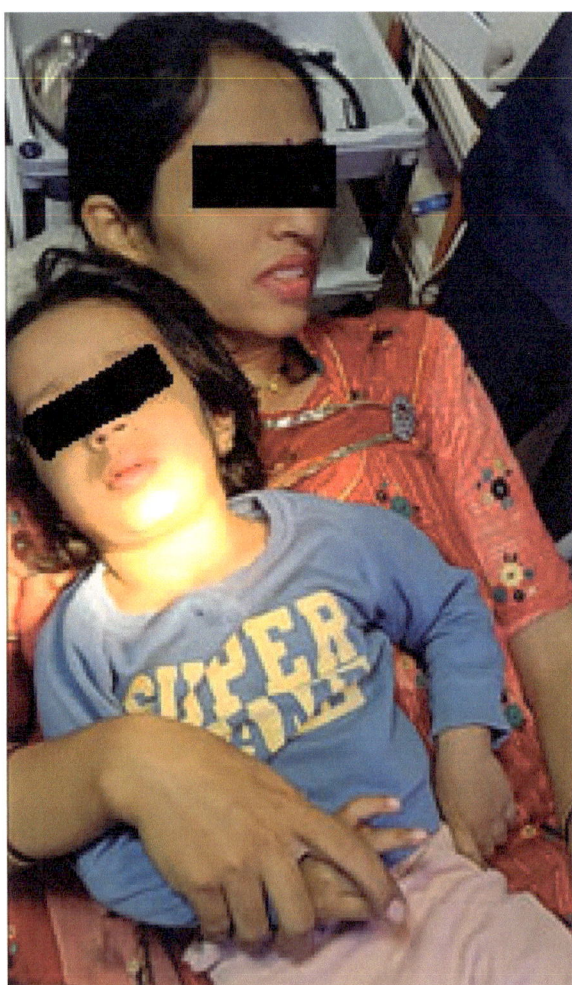

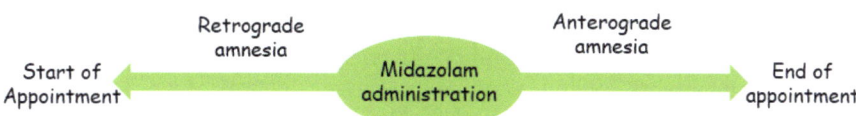

Fig. 4.4   Anterograde and retrograde amnesia

analgesic properties in midazolam. But, post procedure, the child may not remember how the soft tissues got numb. This property of lack of recall after administration of midazolam is called anterograde amnesia. But midazolam does not cause retrograde amnesia. So, if a difficult venipuncture attempt was done in the child before midazolam was administered, the child will remember the difficult episode. The concept is explained in Fig. 4.4.

In the event of the pre-cooperative child requiring longer and multiple operative procedures, general anesthesia becomes the most predictable option.

4.4.4.4   Frankl Definitely Negative Behavior - - 3
(Disruptive/uncontrolled/hysterical/combative behavior stemming either from severe objective fear or from specific debilitating conditions like intellectual and developmental disability)

Traits of Frankl Definitely Negative Behavior - - 3
This group of children are very obvious to recognize. They are potentially cooperative, usually aged between 3 and 6 years. The tantrum or crying usually starts at the reception area, even before the child enters the operatory. The child resists even entering the operatory and has to be forced inside. The child physically lashes out and flails her/his extremities accompanied by loud crying. The behavior of the children is usually due to a real fear traced back to a very traumatic dental or medical experience or previous hospitalization. There is no opportunity for establishment of a two-way communication. The clinician has to recognize that the child has real or severe fear in this case and should refrain from any aggressive posturing or voice modulation.

The other group of children who "*may*" display this behavior are children with intellectual and developmental disabilities (IDD). The severity of their systemic condition prevents establishment of a two-way communication with the clinician. We emphasize on the word "*may*" here because not all children with IDD will display - - 3 behavior.

Behavior Guidance Template for Frankl Definitely Negative Behavior - - 3

Pharmacological Management Plan for *Emergency* Procedures in Children Displaying - - 3 Behavior
Emergency treatment in the above children (subject to medical clearance) can be accomplished with the intramuscular administration (IM) of midazolam at 0.15–0.2 mg/kg body weight [13–15]. In a disruptive child or a child with

disabilities, intramuscular midazolam can be a very useful behavior management tool [16]. Intranasal midazolam is also a very effective tool in special care dentistry [17]. The intranasal (IN) midazolam dosage for emergency care is 0.3–0.4 mg/kg body weight. Intranasal dexmedetomidine (*2 mcg/kg body weight*) can also be an option in older children (weighing more than 25 kgs) considering its availability in 100 mcg/ml ampoules. This leads to very small volumes of the drug that will need to be administered intranasally. The IM/IN administration can be administered with minimal restraint to deposit the entire calculated dose, predictably to the child. The short sedation window created can be used to render the emergency treatment to the child. Protective stabilization with a papoose board or pedi-wrap along with a molt prop will likely be required. The child may still cry or resist treatment. But the brief sedation window along with the protective stabilization will allow local anesthetic administration and completion of the emergency dental procedure. The anterograde amnesia provided by midazolam is an added advantage in these already frightened children [18]. The reader is referred to Chap. 5 for details on the technique of IM/IN drug administration.

Pharmacological Management Plan for *Elective* Procedures in Children Displaying - - 3 Behavior

Children in this category with limited treatment needs or requiring *short procedures*, for example, a pulpotomy and a Hall crown [10] or an extraction of a permanent molar, can be treated under deep sedation with an open airway. The reader is referred to Chap. 8 for a detailed discussion on the concepts of deep sedation and general anesthesia.

Open airway is a situation where no airway adjunct like an endotracheal tube or a laryngeal mask airway (LMA) will be protecting the glottis. A nasal cannula will supply 100% oxygen along with a nasopharyngeal airway. A moist throat pack will be present. Intense monitoring and airway assistance as required will be provided by the anesthesiologist. Potent drugs like ketamine, fentanyl, propofol and gaseous anesthetics among other drugs will be used in various combinations by the anesthesiologist to achieve deep sedation, which is essentially an ultra-light plane of general anesthesia [19, 20]. The monitoring, the infrastructure, and the personnel required are on par with general anesthesia requirements [21]. This plane easily overrides the fear and the disruptive behavior of the child. The clinician though should be conscious of the obtunded cough and swallowing reflex in deep sedation with an open airway predisposing the child to laryngospasm from the foreign bodies (debris, water, saliva, blood, etc.) generated during the dental operative procedures. Water should be judiciously used in these cases along with the use of rubber dam [22]. The rubber dam should also be carefully placed especially when the entire mandibular arch is isolated. Full mandibular arch rubber dam isolation may further exacerbate respiratory compromise by pushing the tongue back and further physically blocking the airway. It is once again emphasized that deep sedation with an open airway is only indicated for limited treatment needs. The rationale of using deep sedation with an open airway is only to obtain the benefit of a lighter plane of anesthesia, facilitating a faster recovery and discharge.

For *long or multiple* procedures, - - 3 children are best treated under general anesthesia with endotracheal intubation. The procedure can be done in the hospital operating room utilizing a combination of anesthetic gases and intravenous drugs. It may also be accomplished in the dental office well-equipped with the recommended infrastructure for general anesthesia using the total intravenous anesthesia (TIVA) technique, teaming with the anesthesiologist.

4.5   Indications of Midazolam in a Nutshell

Understanding midazolam along with its limitations is the key to outlining its indications. Midazolam, when used where indicated, leads to successful outcomes consistently. This in turn adds another effective behavior guidance tool into the clinician's armamentarium. The vice versa is also true. Overestimating the capabilities of midazolam and using it as a hit-and-trial drug to overcome hysterical behavior in children leads to paradoxical reactions and failure. This in turn results in the clinician losing confidence in the drug. So reemphasizing again that moderate sedation with midazolam is most effective only when combined with sound techniques of communicative behavior guidance and local anesthesia, this chapter ends by drawing a practical list of indications for midazolam based on the Frankl rating of the child. The concept is represented in Fig. 4.5.

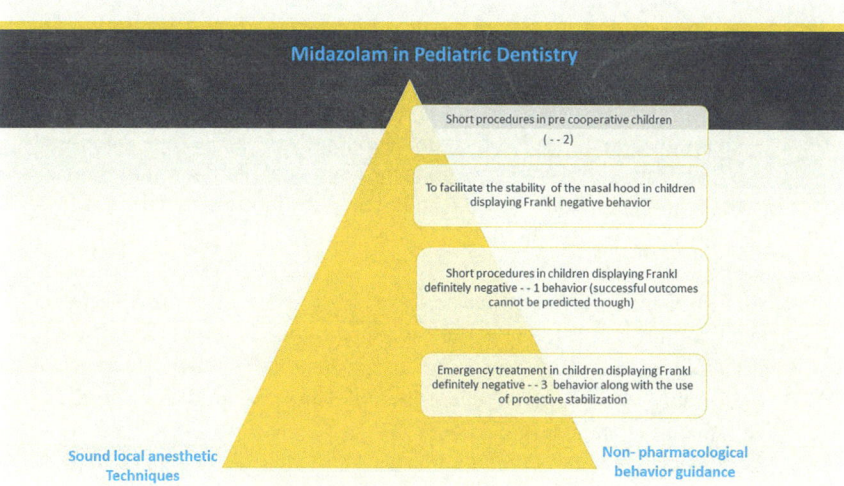

Fig. 4.5 Indications of midazolam in Pediatric Dentistry

Clinically Relevant Points

1. The behavior guidance templates suggested for each Frankl category in this chapter do not intend to oversimplify child management. These templates should be used only as a guide and not be considered a "one glove fits all" solution. There may be more clinical presentations of child behavior under each Frankl category. The behavior may also overlap between Frankl categories, and the clinician must sense subtle nuances in behavior and flexibly use the strategies based on the presenting clinical situation.

2. The clinician must recognize the Frankl positive rating trait and proceed carefully. One unpleasant episode may result in sudden loud crying. The behavior rating could quickly change to Frankl negative or definitely negative.

3. Children displaying Frankl negative behavior *do not* actively resist treatment but will "whine" or "cry" throughout the treatment.

4. In the above category of children, oral midazolam within prescribed doses will calm the child, decrease anxiety, and create an environment where the child will be more receptive to the clinician's communicative efforts. The nasal hood followed by inhalation sedation can also be introduced under its influence.

5. Frankl definitely negative behavior has several clinical presentations. It is a broad category, which does not provide sufficient clinical information about the specifics of the negative behavior.

6. These children can be further subdivided as children displaying:

   - Defiant, stubborn, or mild fearful behavior stemming either from subjective fear or overindulgent parenting.
   - Pre-cooperative behavior.
   - Disruptive/uncontrolled/hysterical/combative behavior stemming either from severe objective fear or from specific debilitating conditions like intellectual and developmental disability.

7. The above three subcategories can be denoted clinically as - - 1, - - 2, and - - 3, respectively.

8. A child displaying - -1 behavior, convinced to cooperate for the dental treatment through voice modulation or parent intervention, would still be very anxious. The clinician should ensure that the treatment is carried out comfortably, using sound techniques of behavior guidance, moderate sedation, and local anesthesia.

9. Short procedures in - - 2 behavior category of children can be predictably accomplished using oral (squirt method of administration) or intranasal midazolam.

10. Emergency treatment for - - 3 behavior category of children can be accomplished with the intramuscular or intranasal administration of midazolam in conjunction with protective stabilization.

11. These children (- - 3 behavior) with limited treatment needs, for example, requiring a short restorative procedure like a pulpotomy and a Hall crown, can be treated under deep sedation with an open airway teaming with an anesthesiologist.

12. Deep sedation and general anesthesia are a continuum, and the terminology or definitions are only academic. In deep sedation, the child is in the Guedel stage 1 of anesthesia or in the ultra-light plane of general anesthesia.

13. For long or multiple procedures, the children displaying - - 3 behavior are best treated under general anesthesia with endotracheal intubation. The procedure can be done in the hospital operating room utilizing a combination of anesthetic gases and intravenous drugs. It may also be accomplished in the dental office well-equipped with the recommended infrastructure for general anesthesia using the total intravenous anesthesia (TIVA) technique, along with an anesthesiologist.

14. In a nutshell, the indications for the use of midazolam in Pediatric Dentistry will be:

    - For short procedures in pre-cooperative children (- - 2)
    - To facilitate the stability of the nasal hood in children displaying Frankl negative behavior
    - For short procedures in children displaying Frankl definitely negative - - 1 behavior (successful outcomes cannot be predicted though)
    - For emergency treatment in children displaying Frankl definitely negative - - 3 children, in conjunction with protective stabilization

15. Midazolam is indicated for an anxious child who is ready to accept treatment. It helps the child cope up with the stress of the dental treatment. It is not strong enough in prescribed dosages to overcome strong resistance in a child who is *not* ready to accept treatment.

References

1. Veerkamp JSJ, Wright GZ. Children's behavior in the dental office. In: Wright GZ, Kupietzky A, editors. Behavior management in dentistry for children. 2nd ed. Wiley Blackwell. p. 23–33.
2. Frankl SN, Shiere FR, Fogels HR. Should the parents remain with the child in the dental operatory? J Dent Child. 1962;29:22–35.
3. Dean AJ. Behavior management. In: Shanthala BM, editor. McDonald and Avery's, dentistry for the child and adolescent, 2nd south Asia edition. Elsevier India; 2019. p. 171–95.
4. Becker DE, Bennett CR. Intravenous and intramuscular sedation. In: Dionne RA, Phero JC, Becker DE, editors. Management of pain and anxiety in the dental office. 1st ed. WE Saunders Company; 2002. p. 235–60.
5. Attri JP, Sharan R, Makkar V, Gupta KK, Khetarpal R, Kataria AP. Conscious sedation: emerging trends in Pe-diatric dentistry. Anesth Essays Res. 2017;11:277–81.

6. Current JL, Unkel JH, Berry EJ, Reinhartz J, Reinhartz D. Comparing behavior outcomes with rubber dam or IsoVac isolation in patients undergoing moderate sedation. J Dent Child (Chic). 2022;89(2):83–7.
7. Nathan JE. Retrospective comparisons of the efficacy and safety of variable dosing of midazolam with and without meperidine for management of varying levels of anxiety of pediatric dental patients: 35 years of sedation experience. J Clin Pediatr Dent. 2022;46(2):152–9. https://doi.org/10.17796/1053-4625-46.2.11.
8. Kher M, Rao A. Lesion management: no removal of carious tissue. In: Kher M, Rao A, editors. Contemporary treatment techniques in pediatric dentistry. Cham, Switzerland: Springer; 2019. p. 99–116.
9. Hesse D, Bonifácio CC, Mendes FM, Braga MM, Imparato JC, Raggio DP. Sealing versus partial caries removal in primary molars: a randomized clinical trial. BMC Oral Health. 2014;14:58. https://doi.org/10.1186/1472-6831-14-58.
10. Innes NPT, Evans DJP. The hall technique as a new method for managing caries in primary molars: is it really a revolution? In: Splieth CH, editor. Revolutions in pediatric dentistry.
11. Kupietzky A, Houpt MI. Midazolam: a review of its use for conscious sedation of children. Pediatr Dent. 1993;15(4):237–41.
12. Payne KA, Coetzee AR, Mattheyse FJ. Midazolam and amnesia in pediatric premedication. Acta Anaesthesiol Belg. 1991;42:101–5.
13. Malamed SF. Intramuscular sedation. In: Sedation: a guide to patient management, 6th ed. St. Louis, MO: Elsevier; 2018, pp. 134–163.
14. Lam C, Udin RD, Malamed SF, Good DL, Forrest JL. Midazolam premedication in children: a pilot study comparing intramuscular and intranasal administration. Anesth Prog. 2005;52(2):56–61. https://doi.org/10.2344/0003-3006(2005)52[56:MPICAP]2.0.CO;2.
15. Shashikiran ND, Reddy SV, Yavagal CM. Conscious sedation--an artist's science! An Indian experience with midazolam. J Indian Soc Pedod Prev Dent 2006 Mar;24(1):7–14. doi: https://doi.org/10.4103/0970-4388.22830.
16. Malamed SF, Quinn CL, Hatch HG. Pediatric sedation with intramuscular and intravenous midazolam. Anesth Prog. 1989;36(4–5):155–7.
17. Drysdale D. The use of intranasal midazolam in a special care dentistry department: technique and cases. Prim Dent J. 2015;4(2):42–8.
18. Nadin G, Coulthard P. Memory and midazolam conscious sedation. Br Dent J. 1997;183(11–12):399–407. https://doi.org/10.1038/sj.bdj.4809520.
19. Ganzberg SI. Deep sedation and GA. In: Wilson S, editor. Oral sedation for dental procedures in children. Berlin: Springer; 2015. p. 157–71.
20. Malamed SF. Fundamentals of general anesthesia. In: Sedation: a guide to patient management, 6th ed. St. Louis, MO: Elsevier; 2018, pp. 407–415.
21. Coté CJ, Wilson S. Guidelines for monitoring and management of pediatric patients before, during, and after sedation for diagnostic and therapeutic procedures. Pediatr Dent. 2019;41(4):259–60.
22. Reed KL, Jo OA. Working with a dentist anesthesiologist. In: Wright GZ, Kupietzky A, editors. Behavior management in dentistry for children. 2nd ed. Wiley Blackwell; 2014. p. 177–84.

Routes of Midazolam Administration

5

5.1 Overview

Midazolam being a versatile drug can be administered through various routes including intravenous, oral, intranasal, intramuscular, rectal, and oral mucosal. This chapter will discuss the advantages and disadvantages of each route. It will also discuss the dosage, equipment, technique of administration, and time for onset of action with each route. Numerous clinical tips for each route are also included in the chapter.

5.2 Background and Objective

The case selection based on pre-operative assessment and the Frankl rating of the child were discussed in the preceding Chaps. 3 and 4. In this chapter, we go forward assuming that the route of midazolam sedation has been finalized for the child. Midazolam being a versatile drug can be administered through various routes including intravenous, oral, intranasal, intramuscular, rectal, and oral mucosal. Let us note here that the duration of clinical action and complete recovery from a single dose of midazolam, regardless of the route of administration, remains in the range of 45–90 minutes and 11–13 hours, respectively. The objective of this chapter will be to enable the reader understand the advantages and disadvantages of the various routes, dosage, time for onset of sedation, and technique of administration. The informed consent and the pre-operative instructions for the parents including the "nil per oral (NPO)" instructions have been discussed in Chaps. 9 and 8.

© The Author(s), under exclusive license to Springer Nature Switzerland AG 2024
A. Rao, S. Tiwari, *Midazolam in Pediatric Dentistry*,
https://doi.org/10.1007/978-3-031-45147-8_5

5.3   Where Should the Sedative Drug Be Administered?

Midazolam, with the exception of the intravenous route, should *not* be administered inside the operatory on the dental chair. This may increase the child's anxiety and initiate an aversion to the operatory and the dental chair. The sedative drug should ideally be administered in a quiet room, in the presence of a parent [1]. Soothing music with a neat but not a loud ambiance is a desirable setting during the latency period (*the period between the administration of the drug and the attainment of clinical levels of sedation, adequate for treatment to start*). Post administration, the child should be discouraged from indulging in active play. This is also a good time to introduce a pulse oximeter to the child. An assistant should observe the child for the onset of sedation and alert the clinician when necessary.

The only exception to this rule is when midazolam is administered intravenously. In this case, midazolam should be administered in the operatory on the supine dental chair. This is because there will not be any latency period and the drug acts almost in real time.

5.4   Volume of Drug Distribution and Midazolam Dosage

The volume of distribution (Vd) of midazolam is high because of its lipophilicity (See Chap. 2). If a drug has a propensity to remain in the plasma post absorption, then it is said to have a low Vd. If a drug has the propensity to leave the plasma for extravascular binding to fat or other tissues, it is said to have a high Vd. Vd is a useful tool to determine the loading dose of a drug. Drugs with a lower Vd can be administered in a lower dosage and vice versa. Figure 5.1 schematically explains the concept.

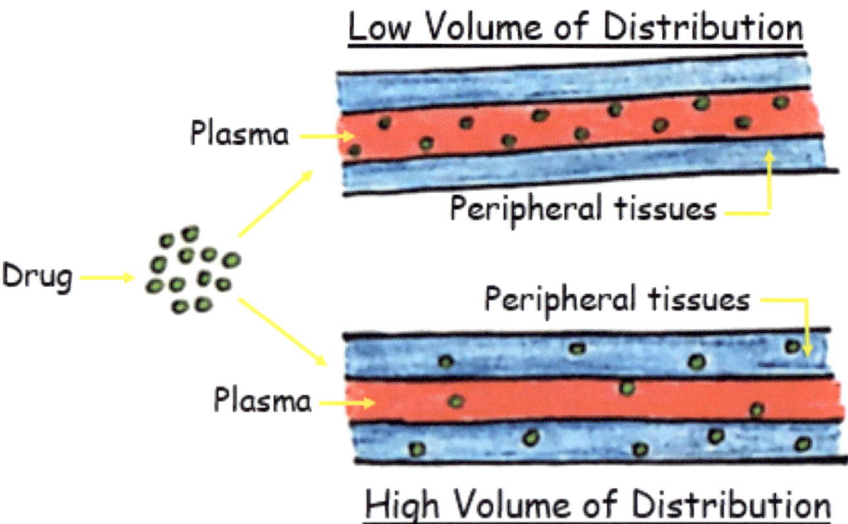

Fig. 5.1 The volume of distribution

This concept may be relevant in determining the drug dosage in overweight or obese children. In overweight/obese children as a general rule, the dose of midazolam should be calculated based on the average weight of children of that age/sex and not on the actual weight of the child (See Sect. 3.4.3 of Chap. 3). This is because, in obese children, midazolam's Vd may further heighten because of increased availability of peripheral adipose tissues [2]. This may lead to a delayed onset of action. To negate this effect in overweight or obese children, a dosage on the higher end of the prescribed range for the selected route is recommended. For example, the prescribed dosage range for oral midazolam is 0.5–0.75 mg/kg body weight. For obese or overweight children, the higher end of the dosage at 0.75 mg/kg body weight may therefore be recommended.

5.5   Intravenous Route of Midazolam Administration

5.5.1   The Practical Role of Intravenous Midazolam in Pediatric Dentistry

The intravenous route is no doubt the most ideal route of administering midazolam for the purpose of moderate sedation. Titration is the main advantage that enhances the safety and effectiveness of this route. The dosage can be titrated predictably with an individually tailored need for moderate sedation. It also provides the ideal mode to administer reversal drugs like flumazenil. Every other route of midazolam administration, be it oral, intranasal, intramuscular, oral mucosal, or rectal, is a compromise on titration. The advantages and disadvantages of other routes are essentially a give and take.

So if the intravenous route is the ideal route, then why do we consider the other routes of administration?

To answer that question, let us first understand the special considerations of Pediatric Dentistry. Pediatric Dentistry deals with the treatment of children from infancy through adolescence. The intravenous route is an ideal route to achieve moderate sedation using midazolam in adolescent children. In prescribed doses, it is in fact one of the safest methods to titrate an anxious adolescent to moderate sedation. The older anxious child calms down as the effect of midazolam takes over. But this won't be the case in a young child. A young child who has undergone venipuncture against her/his approval will try to further fight the effects of midazolam and may end up even more agitated. This is termed a paradoxical reaction. This happens because midazolam is a moderate sedation drug, which is intended for anxiolysis. The use of midazolam intravenously at prescribed dosages *will not* be potent enough to override the fear of the young child. The agitated child will require deep sedation to override her/his fears. In addition to venipuncture, the use of intravenous sedation in a young child comes with many other challenges including small veins, requirement of an anesthesiologist, and intense monitoring. So, if moderate sedation is the goal as required in a young anxious child, midazolam administered via any of the other non-invasive or non-titratable routes with or without inhalation sedation will do the job.

If the objective is deep sedation, it can be better accomplished with other intravenous drugs specific to the purpose like propofol, fentanyl or analogs, or ketamine either alone or in combinations. These drugs in the hands of an anesthesiologist will predictably achieve deep sedation in smaller doses compared to midazolam.

But establishing an intravenous line and learning to start a continuous intravenous infusion is still an important emergency skill that must be learnt by the clinicians practicing sedation in children.

5.5.2   Advantages [3]

- The onset of action is rapid, within 20–25 seconds, taking the drug from the hand where it is administered to the heart and then to the brain. This allows titration where the drug dosage can be customized to each child depending on the sedative effect they display. Recovery is also faster with this route.
- The patent vein available in this technique allows for administration of emergency and reversal drugs like flumazenil.
- A continuous intravenous infusion keeps the child (under NPO) hydrated, in case of long procedures.
- The side effects associated with nausea and vomiting are also less with intravenous sedation. The gag reflex, which is common in children, is also diminished through this route.
- There is very reliable anterograde amnesia with intravenous midazolam.

5.5.3   Disadvantages

- The primary disadvantage in children is the necessity of a venipuncture. This procedure is more challenging due to the proportional smaller veins of children compared to adults.
- The child will very often require premedication through a non-titratable route, like the intramuscular or intranasal route, to tolerate the venipuncture.
- Establishing an intravenous line is a skilled procedure that requires regular practice.
- A continuous intravenous infusion requires additional equipment.
- Because it has a rapid onset of action almost in real time, the potential for adverse effects also increases. Hence, it requires an anesthesiologist for administration and monitoring.

5.5.4   Equipment for Intravenous Infusion [4]

5.5.4.1 Intravenous Infusion Solution (Fig. 5.2)

Lactated Ringer's solution, sterile water for injection, 5% dextrose in water, and sodium chloride injection are the commonly available infusion solutions packaged

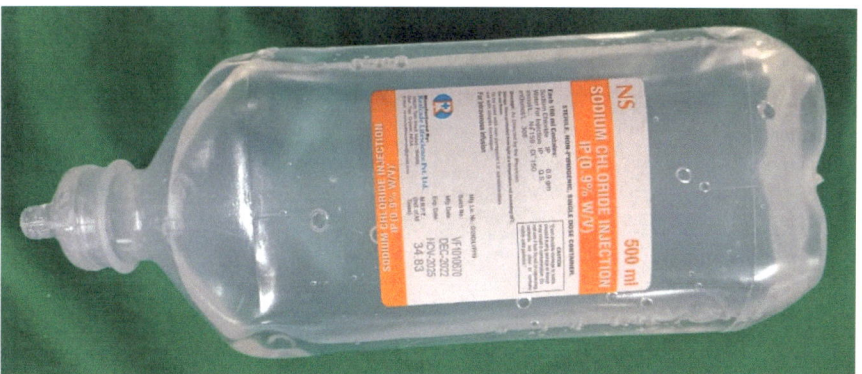

Fig. 5.2 Intravenous infusion solution

in plastic bags. A 500 mL bag is adequate for the dental procedures. The intravenous tubing connects into the intravenous bag.

5.5.4.2 Intravenous Tubing (Fig. 5.3a)

The intravenous tubing carries the infusion solution from the bag to the patient. It has the following parts:

- Piercing pin (Fig. 5.3b): It is the part of the intravenous tubing that is inserted into the intravenous bag.
- Drip chamber (Fig. 5.3b): Immediately below is a clear flexible chamber called the drip chamber. Its main purpose is to prevent air bubbles from entering the tubing. If empty, then each drop of intravenous infusion solution that falls into the drip chamber can potentially create an air bubble that can enter the intravenous tubing. This is prevented by ensuring that the drip chamber is always half-full with the intravenous infusion solution, during its administration to the patient (Fig. 5.3c).
- Drip chambers can be of a macro-dip or micro-drip (pediatric) type. The macro-drip type commonly generates 10–20 drops/mL of the infusion solution. The micro-drip (pediatric) type generates 60 drops/mL. This slows down the rate of infusion, thereby preventing overhydration in a pediatric patient.
- Flow adjustment knob (Fig. 5.3d): This regulates the flow rate from the infusion solution bag into the drip chamber. The controller is rolled that either squeezes or releases the intravenous tubing to regulate the flow rate of the intravenous infusion solution. For example, if a macro-drip generating 20 drops/mL is used, the flow rate can be set to 20 drops/minute using the flow adjustment knob. This translates to an infusion solution flow rate of 1 mL/minute or 60 mL/hour. So, in this case, a 250 mL infusion bag will last for approximately 4 hours.
- Needle adaptor (Fig. 5.3e): It is found at the end of the intravenous tubing. It attaches to the intravenous cannula, which is already inserted into the patient's vein.

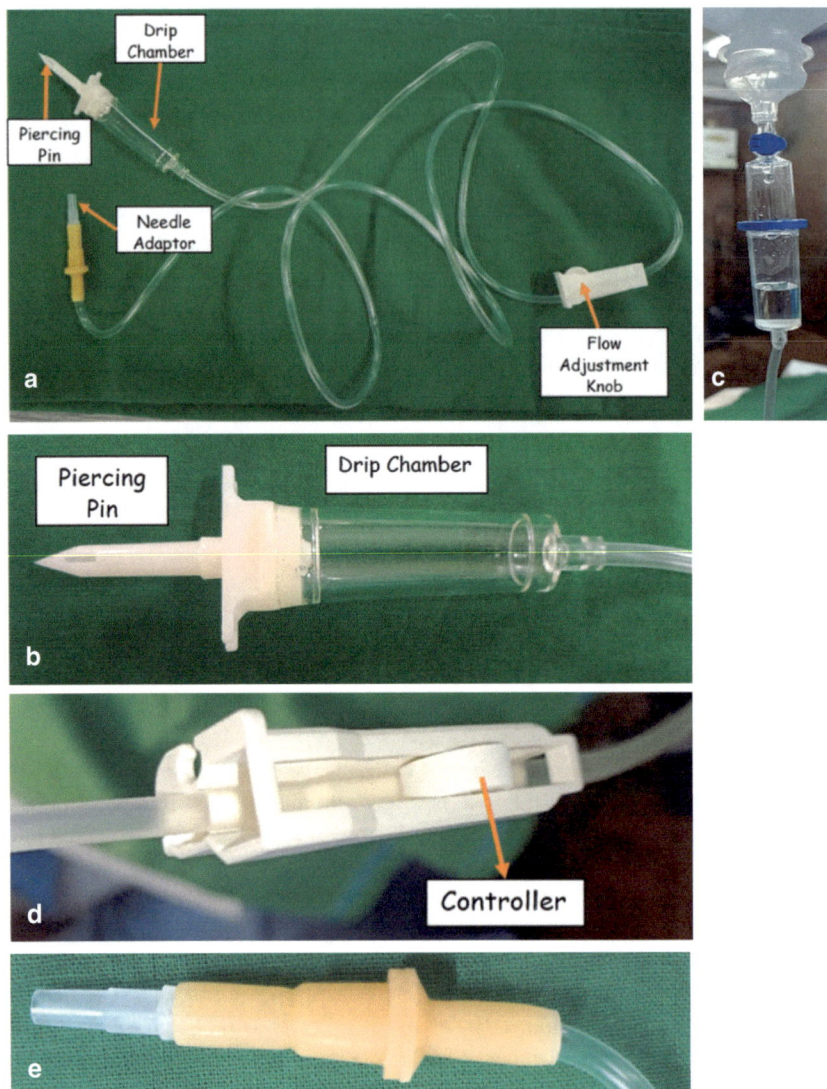

Fig. 5.3 (**a**) The intravenous tubing. (**b**) The piercing pin and the drip chamber. (**c**) The drip chamber partially filled. (**d**) Flow adjustment knob. (e) The needle adaptor

5.5.4.3 Intravenous Cannula

Let us first understand the anatomy of the intravenous cannula by discussing the concept of the "introducer" and the "catheter." The needle called the "introducer" has a radiopaque "catheter" closely adapted over it (Fig. 5.4a–c). The length of the catheter is slightly shorter than the introducer. The introducer is called so because it "introduces" the "catheter" into the vein. The introducer initially penetrates the vein. The catheter is then pushed into the vein and the introducer is removed. The needle adapter of the intravenous tubing is attached to the cannula, and the catheter

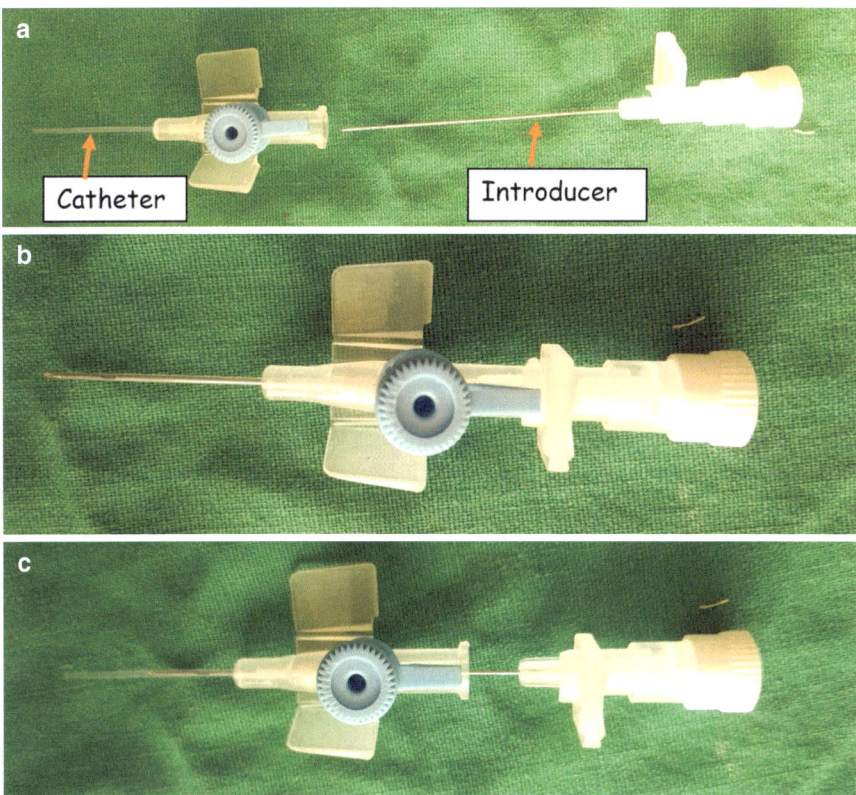

Fig. 5.4 (**a**) The introducer and the catheter. (**b**) Catheter closely adapted over the introducer. (**c**) Introducer partially withdrawn from the catheter

Fig. 5.5 Color coding of intravenous cannulas

Size	Color	Use
14G	Orange	In trauma situations
16G	Gray	Large volume infusions in surgeries
18G	Green	Blood transfusions
20G	Pink	Medications, hydration and routine therapy
22G	Blue	Small veins: pediatric or elderly
24G	Yellow	Fragile veins: pediatric or elderly

is secured with a tape. The detailed process is discussed in Sect. 5.5.5.2 on venipuncture.

The needles used in the intravenous cannula can range from 14 gauge to 24 gauge and are color coded [5] (Fig. 5.5). The lower the gauge number, the larger will be the diameter of the needle lumen.

5.5.4.4 Other Equipment and Materials

1. An intravenous stand is required such that the bag is hung at a level above the patient's heart (Fig. 5.6).
2. A tourniquet is any device that prevents the return of venous blood into the heart but at the same time does not impede arterial supply into the limb. It helps engorging the veins to aid in easy identification and venipuncture (Fig. 5.7a, b).

Fig. 5.6 Intravenous stand

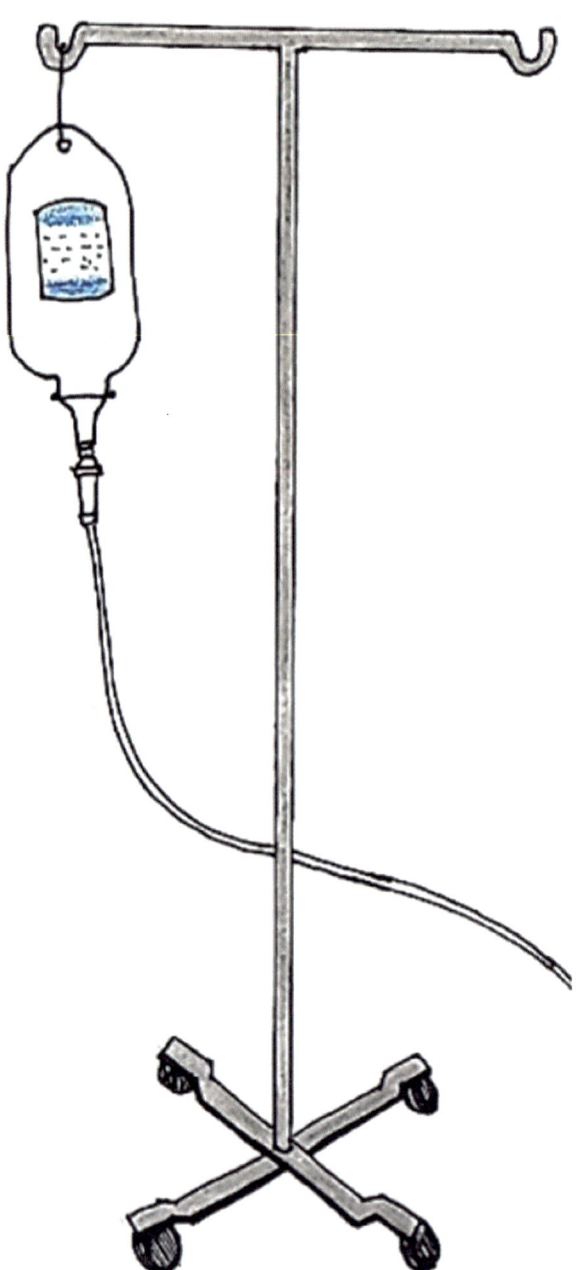

Fig. 5.7 (**a**, **b**) Tourniquet

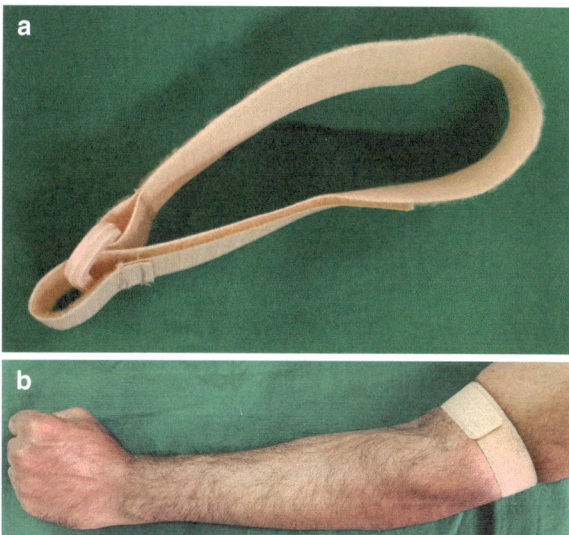

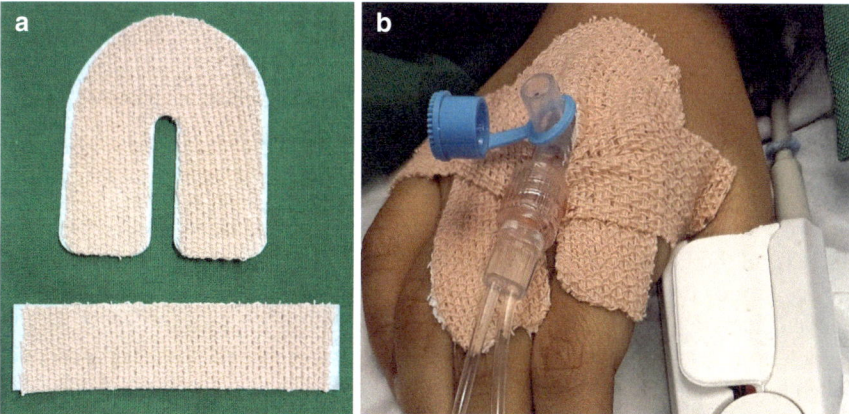

Fig. 5.8 (**a**, **b**) IV cannula adhesive bandage

3. The IV cannula adhesive bandage is used to secure the catheter over the vein (Fig. 5.8a, b).
4. Gauze wipes moistened with isopropyl alcohol are also needed to clean the skin before venipuncture.

5.5.4.5 Readying the IV Infusion Solution Bag and the IV Tubing

The controller on the flow adjustment knob of the intravenous tubing is rolled to a closed position before attaching it to the intravenous infusion solution bag. This is to prevent escape of the intravenous solution on attachment of the intravenous tubing to the solution bag.

The cover on the piercing pin of the intravenous tubing is removed. The piercing pin is firmly attached into the intravenous bag. The bag is now suspended on the intravenous stand.

The drip chamber on the intravenous tubing is squeezed and released alternatively to draw fluid from the bag and fill halfway into the drip chamber.

The controller on the flow adjustment knob is now released to let fluid from the bag flow all the way to the end of the tubing. This is done to remove any air bubbles through the length of the tubing. It is then closed. The intravenous infusion bag and tubing are now ready for use.

5.5.5   Administration

5.5.5.1 Site of Administration [6]
The dorsum of the hand (Fig. 5.9a) is a safe area for venipuncture because the arteries are all located on the palmer surface of the hand. The dorsal venous network on the dorsum of the hand is superficial and is easily located. The water solubility of midazolam allows the clinician to administer it into these small veins safely unlike diazepam.

The ventral aspect of the forearm is also a good area for venipuncture in children with large veins (basilic, cephalic, and median veins) present (Fig. 5.9b).

The above two sites do not need to be immobilized as would be required during venipuncture of the antecubital fossa or the wrist during sedation procedures.

5.5.5.2 Venipuncture [7, 8]
Before we discuss the technique of venipuncture, let us familiarize ourselves with the parts of the IV cannula (Fig. 5.10).

The arm of the patient is allowed to hang freely below the heart level to allow venous blood to pool into the veins.

A tourniquet is applied on the arm above the antecubital fossa. The patient is asked to open and close her/his hands into a fist till the veins appear distended. At

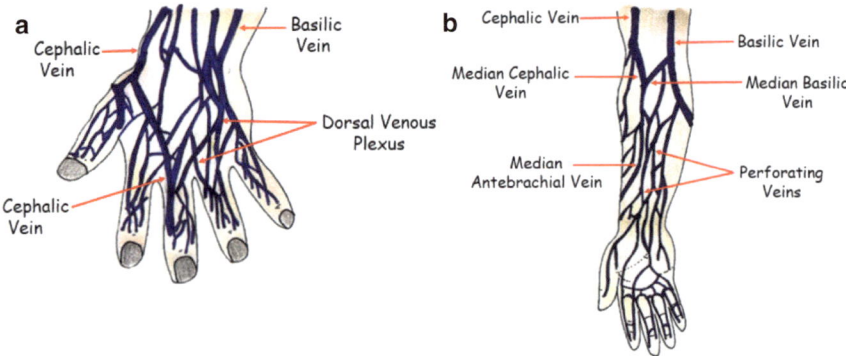

Fig. 5.9 (**a**, **b**) The dorsum and the ventral aspect of the forearm

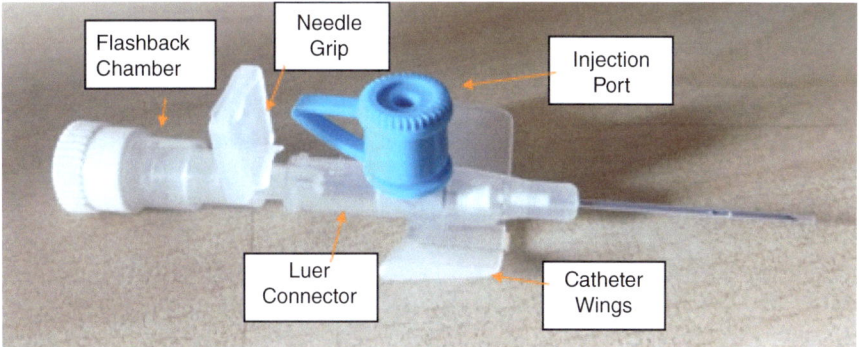

Fig. 5.10 Parts of the IV cannula

this point, the fist should remain closed till venipuncture is completed. Rubbing the skin over the veins or slight tapping can further increase venous distension. The area selected for venipuncture is cleaned with alcohol wipes and dried. The intravenous cannula is placed at a 30° angle to the vein with the bevel of the needle facing up. The skin over the vein is pulled taut with the non-dominant hand. The introducer on the intravenous cannula penetrates the skin and enters the vein. Blood is seen in the "flashback chamber" of the intravenous cannula on vein penetration. This is called the primary flashback. The introducer is further pushed a few millimeters more into the lumen of the vein. Now the "needle grip" of the introducer is stabilized with the non-dominant hand, and the catheter is advanced into the vein slowly without resistance. The "wings" are used to push the catheter into the veins. Blood should be seen moving up the catheter. This is called the secondary flashback. Advance the catheter fully into the vein. Please note that the introducer stays in its place and only the catheter moves forward into the lumen of the vein. Now the tourniquet is removed. The introducer is withdrawn, and the tip of the catheter is occluded within the vein, and the assistant quickly adapts the needle adapter of the intravenous tubing to the "Luer connector" of the catheter and starts the flow of the intravenous solution. The catheter is stabilized initially at the wings with a sterile dressing. An IV cannula adhesive bandage then secures the catheter and the tubing.

5.5.5.3 Dosage
The dosage is 0.025 to 0.1 mg/kg/dose to a maximum of 2 mg/dose titrated to the desired clinical effect. The dosage may be repeated once in 2–3 minutes if needed. The maximum cumulative dose should not exceed 6 mg [9].

5.5.5.4 Technique of Administration [10]
IV midazolam is administered with the 1 mg/mL concentration. The infusion solution flow rate is increased to dilute the drug, keep the vein patent, and prevent localized irritation to the veins. A 0.2 mL test dose is first administered. After 20 s, midazolam is titrated at the rate of 1 mL/min. Administer 0.5 mg over 30 s and wait for a minute before administering further. Slowly titrate at this rate to ideal

moderate sedation. During titration, a common mistake made by the clinician is that titration is stopped at the first visible change in the level of the consciousness of the patient. This leaves the patient very often under-sedated. The ideal level of moderate sedation at which to stop titration is a learning curve perfected with experience. The objective signs of sedation signifying the onset of clinically active sedation include:

- Distant look and less active
- Delayed eye movement
- Unable to stand or sit unaided
- Slurred speech
- Light sleep

The clinical signs and symptoms of ideal moderate sedation will further be described in Chap. 7. Once ideal moderate sedation is achieved, the flow rate of the infusion solution is decreased to a drop every 5–10 seconds. The child can receive 100% oxygen via the nasal hood throughout the procedure.

5.5.6   Onset of Action

The onset of action is in almost real time within 30 seconds to a minute taking the drug from the hand where it is administered to the heart and then to the brain. Though the sedation begins to wane in about 30 minutes time, it is adequate for an hour's appointment under local anesthesia and does not require a second titration.

5.6   The Concept of "Titration by Appointment" for Other Routes

The titration of the drug to effective clinical sedation is not possible with any of the routes of midazolam administration except the intravenous route as discussed. Hence, before we discuss the other routes, let us understand a concept called "titration by appointment." Here, a "bolus recommended dosage" of the drug is administered according to the weight of the child. If the dosage of the sedative drug proves ineffective in the said appointment, then a higher dosage is used in the subsequent appointment [11]. Thus, the drug dosage is individualized over a couple of appointments rather than administering an additional dosage in the same appointment.

5.7   The Oral Route of Midazolam Administration

The oral route is the oldest and the most commonly used route of drug administration. It is especially very favorable for children due to the discomfort associated with other routes [12]. Midazolam is very compatible administered orally. In fact, evidence finds oral midazolam to be more effective than other conscious sedation agents in children undergoing dental treatment [13].

5.7.1 The NPO and the Oral Route

"Nil per oral" (NPO) or the recommended fasting instruction has added significance with the oral route. It is required with the oral route not only to prevent vomiting and potential aspiration but also for the reliable and faster absorption of the drug. The concept is as follows. The small intestine is the primary site of absorption of drugs. So, it is important to get the drugs through the oral cavity, esophagus, and stomach into the small intestine as quickly as possible. Food present in the stomach significantly slows down the gastric emptying time. So it is very important to administer oral midazolam on an empty stomach.

> Gastric emptying time is the time taken for a substance to be expelled from the stomach into the small intestine.

5.7.2 Advantages

- A very economical route of drug administration, with no special armamentarium required.
- The lack of injection or discomfort makes it an attractive proposition in children.
- The incidence and severity of adverse effects are less in this route because it enters the blood stream slowly via the gastrointestinal tract. This assumes that the "single drug-single dose" rule has been followed and does not apply to combinations of oral drugs. See Chap. 8.
- Parents and children's familiarity in administering and accepting drugs, respectively, through the oral route, makes it less intimidating and a very convenient route of sedative drug administration.

5.7.3 Disadvantages

- Even with careful administration, expectoration is a possibility [12].
- The onset of action of the drugs given orally is slower, compared to the parenteral route.
- Titration of the drug to effective clinical sedation is not possible with the oral route.
- A relatively long latency period will be present before the sedative effect of the drug is visible.

> Latency period is the time occurring between the administrations and the onset of clinical action of the drug.

The degree of sedation may vary among individuals, even those with the same weight or body surface area, due to various factors like the presence of food or the emotional makeup of the child. In a very anxious child, there may be delayed and unreliable absorption of the sedative drug [14]. This may also explain why the sedative drug may prove ineffective in a very anxious or fearful child.

Bioavailability of the drug with the oral route will be less because of the hepatic first-pass effect. The drugs administered orally are first taken by the hepatic portal system into the liver before it is absorbed into the systemic circulation. The liver enzymes inactivate some portions of the drug. The bioavailability of oral midazolam is roughly 36% [9]. Thus, a larger dose/kg body weight is required for the oral route compared to the parenteral routes.

> Parenteral route refers to the administration of drugs by bypassing the gastrointestinal system.

5.7.4 Dosage

The dosage for oral midazolam is 0.5–0.75 mg/kg body weight depending on the child temperament [15]. The maximum dose should not exceed 20 mg [9].

5.7.5 Administration

5.7.5.1 Preparation of the Oral Midazolam Solution

Oral midazolam syrup is commercially available as a 2 mg/mL syrup. But these commercial formulations administered in lower dosages are ideally suited for sedation in a non-stressful environment. For procedural sedation of an anxious child in a stressful environment like the dental office, higher dosages will be required. Higher dosages of lower concentration formulations like 2 mg/mL convert to larger volumes, which an anxious child may not accept orally, possibly leading to expectoration or vomiting. So the higher dosages have to be administered in smaller volumes in a pediatric dental scenario. Hence, the more concentrated 5 mg/mL injectable formulation, available in ampules, is well suited for oral sedation in a dental setup (Fig. 5.11).

The solution is extemporaneously prepared by mixing the injectable drug with an equal amount (1:1) of a palatable flavoring agent [16]. Various flavoring agents have been used including acetaminophen syrup, fruit juices, fizzy drinks, and glucose solution. But, as a general rule, oral drugs administered as an aqueous solution are better absorbed compared to a thicker solution like a syrup [11]. But the use of antacids containing sodium citrate or 10% sodium citrate solutions as masking agents is said to increase drug acceptance and produce a faster and deeper level of sedation [17, 18]. Commercially available intravenous midazolam has a pH of 3–3.6. The addition of sodium citrate raises the pH to 4–4.5. At this pH, the imidazole ring of midazolam closes, thereby making it lipophilic. The increased lipid solubility helps

Fig. 5.11 The 5 mg/mL ampule of midazolam

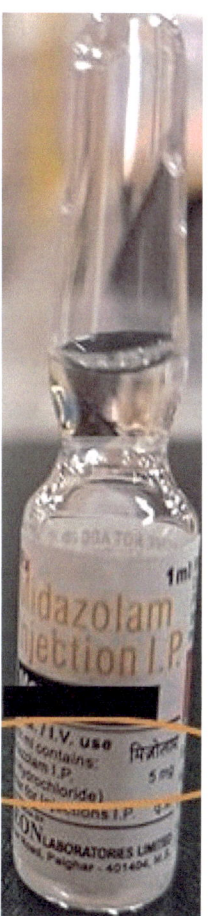

accelerate its absorption across the lipid-rich gastrointestinal membrane into the vascular system.

Also see Chap. 2 for a better understanding of this concept.

Grapefruit juice specifically is not recommended as a flavoring agent. It contains cytochrome P450 3A4 inhibitors (CYP3A4). CYP3A4 is found in the intestine and liver. In the intestine, CYP3A4 aids in absorption of midazolam. So its inhibition leads to decreased absorption and prolonged onset of action of the drug. Of more concern is its consequence in the liver. CYP3A4 in the liver breaks down midazolam into its inactive metabolite. Grapefruit solution containing the inhibitor will prevent this metabolism, resulting in a decreased first-pass metabolism of midazolam in the liver. This results in increased bioavailability of the drug, possibly leading to oversedation [19].

Midazolam is also available as 7.5 mg tablets. But a standard dose like a 7.5 mg tablet may not be ideal in a child where individual doses have to be tailor-made depending on the level of anxiety of the child.

5.7.5.2 Technique of Administration

The oral midazolam solution prepared, is administered to the child by the clinician or parent. The smaller volume of the solution prepared through the 5mg/ml formulation allows it to be administered all at once. This is important because, in spite of the flavoring, the medicine will leave a disagreeable aftertaste. The administration can be followed by a small sip of water to mask the taste. Sipping of the solution should be avoided because the child may refuse further medicine if the taste is unpleasant.

If the child is very anxious and the clinician expects the child to expectorate the medicine, then the squirt method can be used. Here, the undiluted 5 mg/mL solution of midazolam is administered at the prescribed dosage by the clinician via a needle-less syringe, with the child partially reclined. The clinician cradles the head of the child, and the parent stabilizes the extremities. The clinician reflects the cheek with her/his non-dominant hand and slips in a finger/thumb between the teeth and the buccal mucosa onto the retromolar pad. The solution is then deposited slowly via the needleless syringe onto the finger/thumb, which then flows to the oropharynx eliciting a swallowing reflex (Fig. 5.12). The solution should never be rapidly deposited into the throat, which may lead to gagging, chocking, or expectoration. If the child does not swallow the medicine and it grows in volume at the oropharyn-geal area, the administration of the drug should be stopped, and the parent should be requested to gently pinch the nose of the child. The child in an attempt to breathe may reflex swallow the medicine. The rest of the solution can then slowly be admin-istered [15]. This procedure can again be followed by few sips of water.

If the child expectorates or vomits the midazolam solution, a second dose should not be administered in the same appointment. The child may have partially swal-lowed some solution, and some amount may have been absorbed from the mucosa. A second dose may lead to possible oversedation.

5.7.6   Onset of Action

Oral midazolam has a latency period before the sedation sets in. Midazolam absorbed from the small intestine enters the hepatic portal system where a percentage of the drug is metabolized by the liver enzymes called the hepatic first-pass effect. From the liver, the rest of the non-metabolized drug is absorbed into the systemic circulation. The time of onset of sedative action is between 20 to 30 minutes [20].

Fig. 5.12 Squirt method of administration

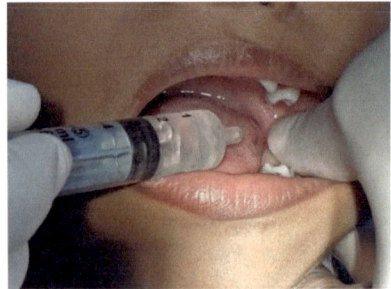

5.8 Intranasal Route of Midazolam Administration

Intranasal administration is a useful alternative to the oral route of midazolam administration in Pediatric Dentistry. It provides a feasible option in children who are reluctant to swallow oral medications. The sedative effects of intranasal midazolam have been shown to be on par with oral midazolam [21].

5.8.1 Advantages Over the Oral Route

- A faster onset of action, usually within 5–10 minutes [21].
- Lack of a long "nil per oral" (NPO): Midazolam administered through the intranasal route showed effective sedation in children who drank milk/cold drink and ate a small meal like a cake within 2 hours of the sedation, compared to those children who were on a 4–6-hours fasting [22]. This is an important advantage considering the children do not have to be fasted for long periods before a stressful dental appointment. The fasting protocol for moderate sedation should have a pragmatic approach because the fluids will not be replenished during the procedure unlike a procedure under general anesthesia. So the potential risk of aspiration should be balanced out with the ill effects of long fasting, namely, hypoglycemia, electrolyte imbalance, and dehydration. The authors though recommend following standard NPO protocols putting safety over everything else. But the child can be administered clear fluids up to 1 hours before the procedure as per the current guidelines of the European Society for Paediatric Anaesthesiology [23, 24]. Volumes upto 3 mL/kg body weight have been recommended [25].
- It is a parenteral technique. The lack of a first-pass metabolism results in an increased bioavailability.
- Less cooperation required from the child compared to the oral route where the child is required to swallow the drug.
- Familiarity of the clinician with the intranasal route is also very important from an emergency point of view. The intranasal route can be used to administer the benzodiazepine reversal agent flumazenil as an emergency measure, when the intravenous route is not available. The dosage is two 100 mcg doses of flumazenil with one dose in each opening of the nares administered through a mucosal atomization device (MAD) [26].

5.8.2 Disadvantages

- It may result in nasal irritation or transient pain resulting in sneezing and spillage around the nostrils.
- The drug may flow into the nasopharyngeal and oropharyngeal mucosa resulting in an unpleasant taste.
- There may be a reverse flow due to excess drug volume resulting in the lack of a predictable dose administered.

- There is potentially a higher incidence of adverse reactions because of the rapid absorption.
- The MAD is also an additional cost to the inventory.
- Protection of the child's eyes will be required.
- The working time may be shorter compared to oral midazolam [11].

5.8.3   Dosage

0.2 mg/kg body weight is the most recommended dosage. But this dose may be adequate as a premedication before additional intravenous sedation or general anesthesia. For procedural sedation only through the intranasal route, higher dosages in the range of 0.3–0.5 mg/kg body weight may be indicated [27].

5.8.4   Administration

5.8.4.1 Different Modes of Intranasal Midazolam Administration

Intranasal midazolam administration was traditionally through a needleless tuberculin syringe, which sprayed the injectable drug into the nares. But this resulted in irritation to the nasal mucosa or the excess drug flowing out, resulting in an unpredictable drug dose administered [21].

Several other commercial formulations are available that provide pre-specified metered doses of the drug (Fig. 5.13).

They are commonly available as 5 and 12.5 mg/mL formulations. They deliver 0.5 mg and 1.25 mg/dose with each press of the device, respectively. The 12.5 mg/mL formulation should be preferred in order to deliver more drug per dose and consequently to reduce the number of times the device is sprayed. The prescribed dosage is split and sprayed equally and alternatively between the nares.

The multiple sprays required into each nares, to achieve the prescribed dosage, is the disadvantage of this mode of administration often leading to behavioral issues with the child. Also, the delivery tip being partially inside the nares during administration, makes it difficult to judge if the dose has been reliably delivered. This is especially true in a crying child.

The mucosal atomization device (MAD) is the ideal way to administer drugs through the intranasal route. It can be attached to a Luer lock syringe (Fig. 5.14).

The pressure on the plunger results in vaporization of the drug into a fine mist as it enters the nose. This minimizes the discomfort of the child to a great deal. The MAD could also form a seal against the nares preventing reverse flow of the drug. Each nostril can accommodate about 1 mL of the drug delivered from the MAD [21]. If the prescribed dosage is beyond 2 mL, then the balance dose is administered, a few minutes later.

Fig. 5.13 Commercially available midazolam intranasal spray

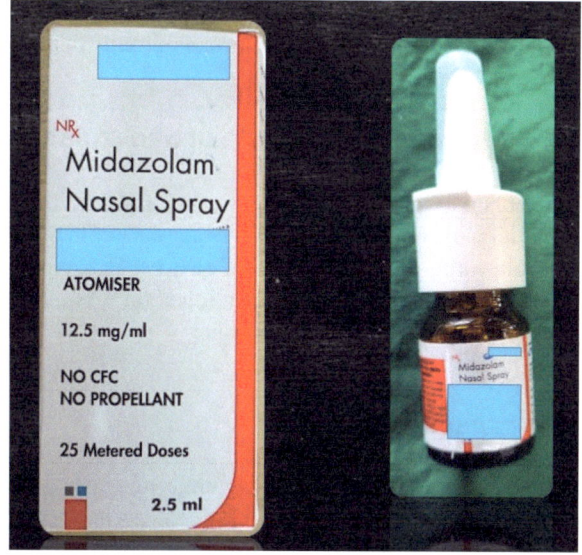

Fig. 5.14 The MAD

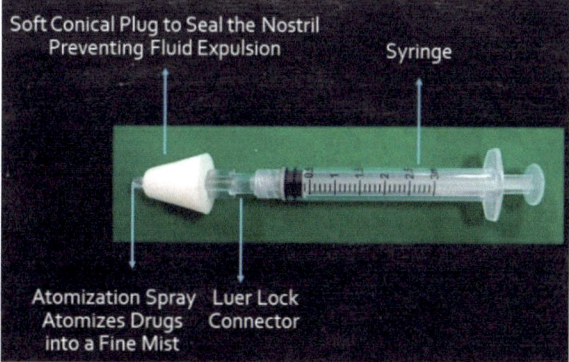

5.8.4.2 Technique of Administration

Regardless of the mode of intranasal delivery, an equal amount of the final dose is administered into each of the nares, with the child in a semi-reclined position and the parent gently restraining the child.

5.8.5 Onset of Action

Absorption into the blood stream happens directly through the blood vessels in the nasal mucosa, thereby avoiding the first-pass metabolism. Though the exact mechanism of action is not understood, it is speculated to be absorbed rapidly into the brain and cerebrospinal fluid through the cribriform plate [12]. There is a rapid onset of action within 5–10 minutes of administration.

5.9 Intramuscular Route of Midazolam Administration

Midazolam in terms of pH and viscosity is safe to be injected intramuscularly. But, in addition to being a useful mode to administer midazolam, the knowledge of intramuscular drug administration can also be lifesaving during an emergency in the dental office. Hence, intramuscular injection techniques are an essential set of skills that should be learnt by all clinicians.

5.9.1 Advantages

- In a disruptive child or a child with disabilities, intramuscular midazolam is a very useful tool [28]. With minimal restraint, the entire calculated dose of midazolam can be predictably given to the child via the intramuscular route. This is one of the major advantages of the intramuscular route compared to the oral or the intranasal route where some drug may potentially be lost, if the child spits or sneezes during administration.
- Since there is no wastage, there is more reliable absorption and a predictable latency period.
- It is also a valuable route for administration of emergency drugs especially in the dental office.
- It retains the advantages of intranasal midazolam like lack of a long NPO, bypassing the hepatic first-pass metabolism, ease of administration, rapid onset of action, and better absorption.
- It can be used as a precursor or premedication to facilitate intravenous sedation or general anesthesia.
- No special equipment is needed.

5.9.2 Disadvantages

- The need of an injection is probably the most obvious disadvantage of the intramuscular route.
- The drug has to be injected deep into the muscle mass where the vascularity is high. This is essential for reliable absorption of the drug. Deposition into the superficial layers of muscles will provide unreliable absorption especially in an anxious child, due to vasoconstriction.

5.9.3   Dosage

0.15–0.2 mg/kg body weight [29]. The maximum should not exceed 10 mg/dose [9].

5.9.4   Administration

5.9.4.1 Site of Administration

The vastus lateralis is the safest region to deposit intramuscular drugs in children. It can accommodate a large volume of the drug before muscle distortion and pain can occur. The border formed by the mid-anterior thigh and the midlateral thigh with one hand width above the knee and below the greater trochanter of the femur (groin) lies the band of muscle available for the injection [30] (Fig. 5.15a,b).

It is considered a safe area because the vital structures like the femoral vessels and the sciatic nerve lie on the mesial and posterior aspects of the thigh. It is the most commonly used muscle for intramuscular injections in children. In an emergency, this site can be used to administer injections through the clothing.

5.9.4.2 Technique of Administration

The area of injection is cleaned with an isopropyl alcohol gauze, moving outward in a circle. The alcohol is allowed to dry before the injection to avoid pushing it into the tissues and the resultant pain. The muscle is held between the thumb and the fingers of the non-dominant hand to raise it, increase the thickness, and make it taut. A 2 mL disposable syringe with a 23 gauge, 1 inch needle is usually used. Standard precautions like ensuring the absence of air bubbles inside the syringe barrel are very important to prevent complications like air embolism. The syringe is held with a dart grasp and inserted 90° into the muscle tissue. No more than three-fourths the length of the needle should enter the muscle tissue to avoid the needle hitting the

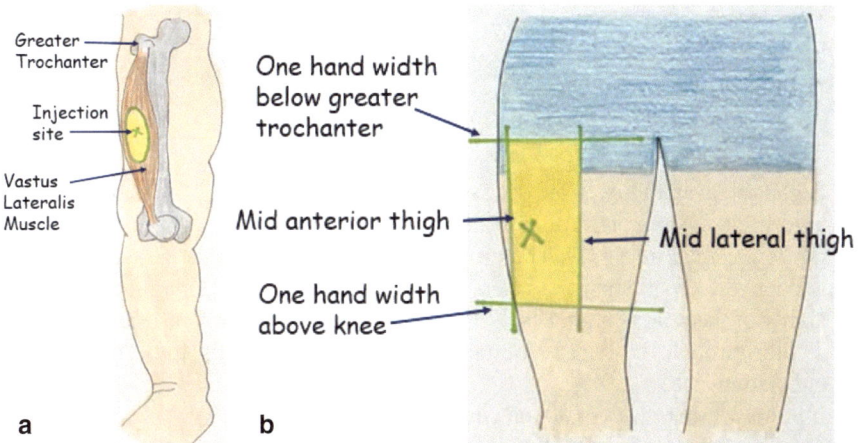

Fig. 5.15 (**a, b**) Landmarks for an injection into the vastus lateralis (lateral view of the right thigh)

femur bone underneath, which can result in pain from periostitis. Aspirate and if negative deposit the drug into the muscle. If aspiration is positive, withdraw the needle and apply pressure on the area. The injection should be slow to prevent pain. The taut muscle should also be loosened as the drug is injected, to prevent its back-flow. A sterile dry gauze is placed on the injection site for a couple of minutes as the needle is withdrawn to prevent bleeding. The needle is then safely disposed. Massage the area to increase the blood supply and thereby the drug absorption.

5.9.5   Onset of Action

10–15 minutes post administration [31, 32].

5.10   Rectal Route of Midazolam Administration

The rectal route does play an important role in some clinical situations like the administration of an analgesic, post dental treatment of children under general anesthesia. It is also a known route for administration of midazolam in Pediatric Dentistry. Unlike diazepam, midazolam has not shown to produce rectal irritation. Many studies have shown rectal midazolam to be very effective in children [33–36].

5.10.1 Advantages

It can be a useful enteral route especially in children who may not be willing candidates for the oral route.

> Enteral route involves the administered drug getting absorbed from the small intestine.

- Higher bioavailability of the drug compared to the oral route. The mechanism of absorption of drugs is similar to that which happens via the oral route from the gastrointestinal tract [37]. The drugs administered through the rectal route also undergo the hepatic first-pass metabolism like the oral route, though the bioavailability of the drug is higher. This could be because of the venous drainage of the rectum through the hepatic portal system and also directly into the systemic circulation.
- It offers a faster onset of action compared to the oral route.
- The needleless administration is an advantage compared to the intramuscular route.
- It also tends to produce less nausea and vomiting.

5.10.2 Disadvantages

- Modesty issues related to rectal administration in the dental office, especially in older children [38].
- A standard NPO time will be required.
- The child should have defecated shortly before the rectal administration of the drug.
- Additional equipment required for drug administration rectally.

5.10.3 Dosage

0.35–0.5 mg/kg body weight [33].

5.10.4 Technique of Administration

Ideally rectally administered drugs should be suppositories, but the injection form of midazolam can be administered through the rectal route. The 5 mg/mL midazolam solution is diluted with saline to a concentration of 2 mg/mL [39]. It is administered inside the anal canal into the rectum of the large intestine (Fig. 5.16). If the volume of the solution to be administered exceeds 10 mL, then the undiluted 5 mg/mL solution is used [39]. The lubricated tip of suitable rectal applicator, rectal catheter, or 14-Fr suction catheter [39] is inserted 5–7 cms into the anal canal to deliver the drug. The buttock cheeks are closed for 5 minutes post administration to prevent loss of the drug.

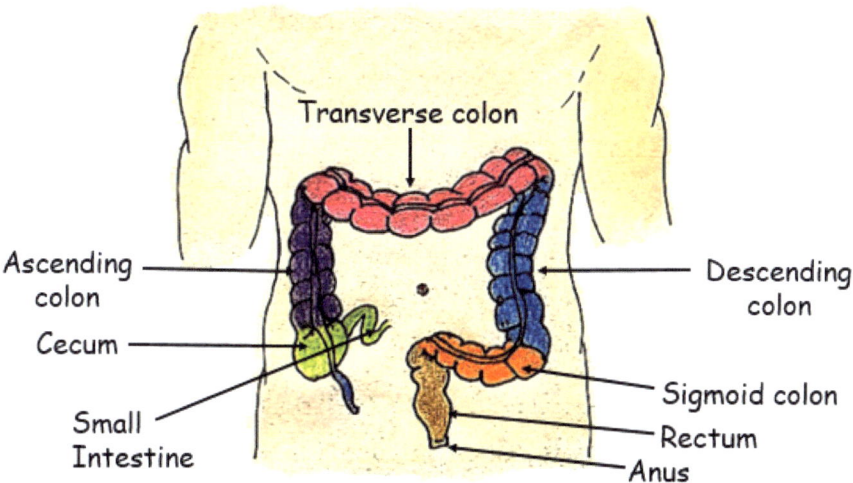

Fig. 5.16 The large intestine

5.10.5 Onset of Action

The treatment can be started within 10 minutes [34].

5.11   Oral Mucosal Route of Midazolam Administration

The oral mucosal delivery of drugs is a well-known route of drug administration. Nitroglycerin for the management of angina pectoris has been administered through this route for over hundred years [40]. Nifedipine for acute hypertensive emergencies and opioids like fentanyl and meperidine for the relief of pain in cancer are other drugs that have been used through this route. Midazolam and triazolam are the benzodiazepines that have been successfully administered through this route.

The sublingual and the buccal tissues are the most common oral mucosal drug delivery routes. The drugs through this route are quickly absorbed through the mucous membranes into the blood stream. Buccal midazolam is now being frequently used for the treatment of seizures [41, 42]. Licensed buccal formulations are now available for this purpose though their efficacy for sedation to facilitate dental treatment in children has not been proven. They are available as prefilled, age-specific oral syringes of 5 mg/mL concentration [41].

5.11.1 Advantages

The oral submucosal route does offer some advantages over the injectable and enteral routes.

• No hepatic first-pass metabolism and hence higher bioavailability.
• Thin oral mucosal lining and a rich vascular supply in the area offers quick absorption of the drug into the systemic circulation and hence a quick onset of action.
• The lack of injection makes it less intimidating for children.
• No special equipment and hence cost-effective.
• Higher acceptance has been shown by children for this route compared to intranasal administration [43, 44].

5.11.2 Disadvantages

• It requires cooperation on part of the child to hold the medicine inside the oral cavity for at least half a minute to ensure sufficient time for sublingual absorption. This limits its use as a sedative route for midazolam, as the drug is intended to be used on anxious children who may not follow instructions.
• The amount of drug absorption could be inconsistent.

5.11.3 Dosage

0.2–0.3 mg/kg body weight [43, 45]. The authors prefer a higher dosage of 0.4–0.5 mg/kg body weight.

5.11.4 Technique of Administration

For sublingual administration, the child is asked to place the tip of the tongue behind the upper anterior teeth. 5 mg/mL formulation is placed under the tongue with a needleless syringe or a mucosal atomization device. The child is asked to close the mouth, but not swallow the drug for 30 seconds, following which the child is asked to swallow the drug [45].

For buccal administration similarly, the needleless syringe or the mucosal atomization device is used to deposit the 5 mg/mL midazolam solution into the mandibular buccal sulci of both the quadrants. The child is encouraged to hold the medication for a few seconds without swallowing it [42].

The commercially available intranasal sprays can also be used off-label (*Kumar A, Personal Communication, June 21, 2022*), through the oral mucosal route (see Sect. 5.8 for details on commercially available intranasal sprays). The 12.5 mg/mL formulation should be preferred in order to deliver more drug per dose and consequently to reduce the number of times the device is sprayed. The device is held vertically into the maxillary arch in the first primary molar region. A small space is kept between the atomizer tip and the vestibule to enable the clinician to see the actual release of the drug with each press of the device (Fig. 5.17).

Fig. 5.17 Oral mucosal delivery with the intranasal midazolam spray

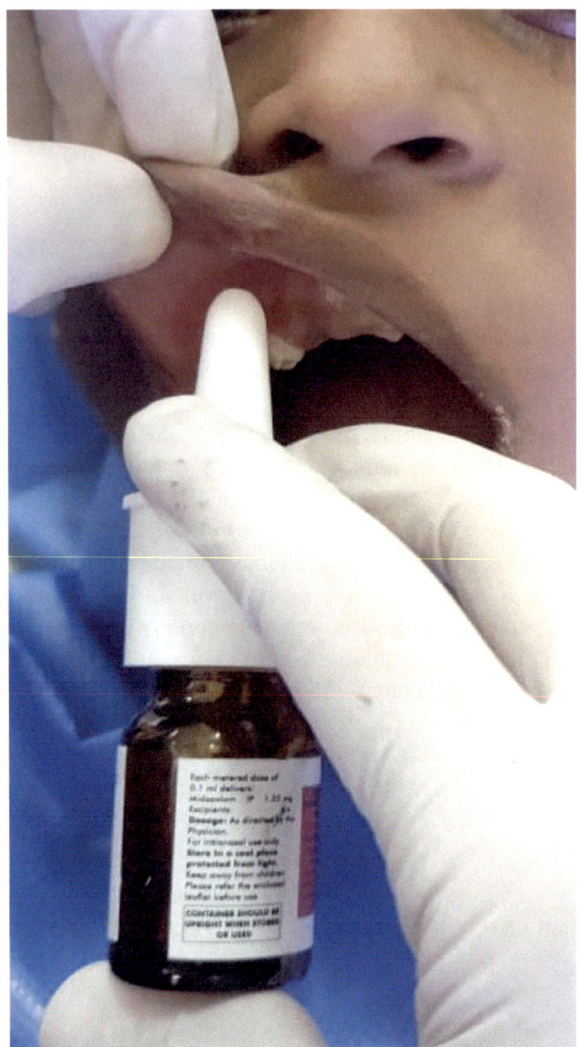

5.11.5 Onset of Action

Ten to twenty minutes post drug administration [45, 46].

Clinically Relevant Points
1. Midazolam should not be administered inside the operatory, which may increase the child anxiety. The only exception to this rule is when midazolam is administered intravenously.

2. "Titration by appointment" is a concept (*for all routes except the intrave-nous route where titration is possible*) where if the dosage of the sedative drug proves ineffective in the said appointment, then a higher dosage can be used in the subsequent appointment.

3. In obese children, midazolam has an increased Vd because of increased affinity to peripheral adipose tissues. Hence, for obese or overweight children, the higher end of the drug dose prescribed for the selected route of administration (*again, not applicable to the intravenous route*) may be indicated.

4. Being a moderate sedation drug, the use of midazolam intravenously will not be enough to override the fear of a young disruptive child.

5. The dorsum of the hand is a safe area for venipuncture because the arter-ies are all located on the palmer surface of the hand.

6. During titration in intravenous midazolam administration, a common mistake made by the clinician is that titration is stopped at the first visible change in the level of the consciousness of the patient. This leaves the patient very often under-sedated. The ideal level of moderate sedation at which to stop titration is a learning curve learnt and perfected with experience.

7. "Nil per oral" (NPO) or the recommended fasting instruction has added significance with the oral route. It is required with the oral route not only to prevent vomiting and potential aspiration but also for the reliable and faster absorption of the drug.

8. Oral midazolam syrup is commercially available as a 2 mg/mL syrup. But the 5 mg/mL injectable formulation available in ampules is better suited for oral sedation in a dental setup.

9. The use of antacids containing sodium citrate or 10% sodium citrate solu-tions used as masking agents is said to increase drug acceptance and pro-duce a faster and deeper level of sedation.

10. The midazolam solution should be administered orally all at once. This is important because, in spite of the flavoring, the medicine will leave a disagreeable aftertaste. Sipping of the solution should be avoided because the child may refuse further medicine if the taste is unpleasant.

11. The intranasal route can also be used to administer the benzodiazepine reversal agent flumazenil as an emergency measure when the intravenous route is not available.

12. The mucosal atomization device (MAD) is the ideal way to administer drugs through the intranasal route.

13. In addition to being a useful mode to administer midazolam, the knowl-edge of intramuscular drug administration can also be lifesaving during an emergency in the dental office.

14. The major advantage of the intramuscular route is that with minimal restraint, the entire calculated dose of midazolam can be predictably given to the child.

15. The vastus lateralis is the safest region to deposit intramuscular drugs in children.
16. Modesty issues related to rectal administration in the dental office especially in older children are a big disadvantage of the rectal route.
17. The disadvantage of the oral mucosal route of midazolam administration is that the child is expected to hold the medication for a few seconds without swallowing it. This limits its use as a sedative route for midazolam, as the drug is intended to be used on anxious children who may not follow instructions.

References

1. Alzahrani AM, Wyne AH. Use of oral midazolam sedation in pediatric dentistry: a review. Pak Oral Dent J. 2012;32(3):444–55.
2. Reves JG, Fragen RJ, Vinik HR, Greenblatt DJ. Midazolam: pharmacology and uses. Anesthesiology. 1985;62(3):310–24.
3. Malamed SF. Intravenous moderate sedation: rationale. In: Sedation: a guide to patient management. 6th ed. St. Louis, MO: Elsevier; 2018. p. 279–84.
4. Malamed SF. Armamentarium. In: In: sedation: A guide to patient management. 6th ed. St. Louis, MO: Elsevier; 2018. p. 285–97.
5. Matt Vera. How to start an IV? 50+ tips & techniques on IV insertion. In: Nurselabs. October 14, 2021. https://nurseslabs.com/how-to-start-an-iv-insertion-tips/ Accessed 6 Nov 2021.
6. Malamed SF. Anatomy for venipuncture. In: Sedation: a guide to patient management. 6th ed. St. Louis, MO: Elsevier; 2018. p. 298–307.
7. Jones O. Intravenous cannulation. In: TeachMeSurgery. September 2, 2018. https://teachmesurgery.com/skills/clinical/cannulation/ Accessed 6 Nov 2021.
8. Malamed SF. Venipuncture technique. In: Sedation: a guide to patient management. 6th ed. St. Louis, MO: Elsevier; 2018. p. 308–18.
9. Midazolam drug monograph. https://www.clinicalkey.com/#!/content/drug_monograph/6-s2.0-403 In: Clinicalkey. Accessed 14 April 2023.
10. Malamed SF. Intravenous moderate sedation: techniques of administration. In: Sedation: a guide to patient management. 6th ed. St. Louis, MO: Elsevier; 2018. p. 359–79.
11. Malamed SF. Oral sedation. In: Sedation: a guide to patient management. 6th ed. St. Louis, MO: Elsevier; 2018. p. 95–119.
12. Lee-Kim SJ, Fadavi S, Punwani I, Koerber A. Nasal versus oral midazolam sedation for pediatric dental patients. J Dent Child (Chic). 2004;71(2):126–30.
13. Ashley PF, Chaudhary M, Lourenço-Matharu L. Sedation of children undergoing dental treatment. Cochrane Database Syst Rev. 2018;12(12):CD003877. https://doi.org/10.1002/14651858.CD003877.
14. Magni G, Cadamuro M, Borgherini G, Mastropaolo G, Di Mario F. Psychological stress and gastric emptying in normal subjects. Psychol Rep. 1991;68(3 Pt 1):739–46. https://doi.org/10.2466/pr0.1991.68.3.739.
15. Wilson S. Protocol. In: Wilson S, editor. Oral sedation for dental procedures in children. Berlin: Springer; 2015. p. 113–39.
16. Goho C. Oral midazolam-grapefruit juice drug interaction. Pediatr Dent. 2001;23(4):365–6.
17. Isik B, Baygin O, Bodur H. Effect of drinks that are added as flavoring in oral midazolam premedication on sedation success. Paediatr Anaesth. 2008;18(6):494–500. https://doi.org/10.1111/j.1460-9592.2008.02462.x.

18. Lammers CR, Rosner JL, Crockett DE, Chhokra R, Brock-Utne JG. Oral midazolam with an antacid may increase the speed of onset of sedation in children prior to general anaesthesia. Pediatr Anesth. 2002;12:26–8. https://doi.org/10.1046/j.1460-9592.2002.00770.x.
19. Kane GC, Lipsky JJ. Drug-grapefruit juice interactions. Mayo Clin Proc. 2000;75(9):933–42. https://doi.org/10.4065/75.9.933.
20. Singh N, Pandey RK, Saksena AK, Jaiswal JN. A comparative evaluation of oral midazolam with other sedatives as premedication in pediatric dentistry. J Clin Pediatr Dent. 2002;26(2):161–4. https://doi.org/10.17796/jcpd.26.2.j714x4795474mr2p.
21. Milnes AR, Wilson S. Alternative to oral sedation. In: Wilson S, editor. Oral sedation for dental procedures in children. Berlin: Springer; 2015. p. 141–55.
22. Al-Rakaf H, Bello LL, Turkustani A, Adenubi JO. Intra-nasal midazolam in conscious sedation of young paediatric dental patients. Int J Paediatr Dent. 2001;11(1):33–40. https://doi.org/10.1046/j.1365-263x.2001.00237.x.
23. Frykholm P, Disma N, Andersson H, Beck C, Bouvet L, Cercueil E, Elliott E, Hofmann J, Isserman R, Klaucane A, Kuhn F, de Queiroz SM, Rosen D, Rudolph D, Schmidt AR, Schmitz A, Stocki D, Sümpelmann R, Stricker PA, Thomas M, Veyckemans F, Afshari A. Pre-operative fasting in children: a guideline from the European Society of Anaesthesiology and Intensive Care. Eur J Anaesthesiol. 2022;39(1):4–25. https://doi.org/10.1097/EJA.0000000000001599.
24. Frykholm P, Disma N, Kranke P, Afshari A. The rationale for the recommendations of the European Paediatric Fasting Guideline: improving paediatric anaesthesia and perioperative medicine. Eur J Anaesthesiol. 2022;39(1):1–3. https://doi.org/10.1097/EJA.0000000000001587.
25. Korkusuz M, Basaran B, Et T, Bilge A, Yarimoglu R, Osmanoglu UO. Gastric emptying times of obese and non-obese school-aged children after preoperative clear fluid intake: a prospective observational study. Paediatr Anaesth. 2023;33:539. https://doi.org/10.1111/pan.14658.
26. Heard C, Creighton P, Lerman J. Intranasal flumazenil and naloxone to reverse over-sedation in a child undergoing dental restorations. Paediatr Anaesth. 2009;19(8):795–7; discussion 798–9. https://doi.org/10.1111/j.1460-9592.2009.03069_1.x.
27. Malamed SF. Sublingual, transdermal and intranasal sedation. In: Sedation: a guide to patient management. 6th ed. St. Louis, MO: Elsevier; 2018. p. 125–33.
28. Malamed SF. Intramuscular sedation. In: Sedation: a guide to patient management. 6th ed. St. Louis, MO: Elsevier; 2018. p. 134–63.
29. Malamed SF, Quinn CL, Hatch HG. Pediatric sedation with intramuscular and intravenous midazolam. Anesth Prog. 1989;36(4–5):155–7.
30. Ebraheim N. Vastus lateralis intramuscular injection—everything you need to know . In: YouTube^IN. June 23, 2018. https://www.youtube.com/watch?v=XFog6uSwbuw Accessed 6 Nov 2021.
31. Lu DP. Intramuscular sedation in dentistry. Compendium. 1991;12(9):628, 630, 632 passim.
32. Lam C, Udin RD, Malamed SF, Good DL, Forrest JL. Midazolam premedication in children: a pilot study comparing intramuscular and intranasal administration. Anesth Prog. 2005;52(2):56–61. https://doi.org/10.2344/0003-3006(2005)52[56:MPICAP]2.0.CO;2.
33. Roelofse JA, van der Bijl P, Stegmann DH, Hartshorne JE. Preanesthetic medication with rectal midazolam in children undergoing dental extractions. J Oral Maxillofac Surg. 1990;48(8):791–7; discussion 797. https://doi.org/10.1016/0278-2391(90)90333-w.
34. Lindh-Strömberg U. Rectal administration of midazolam for conscious sedation of uncooperative children in need of dental treatment. Swed Dent J. 2001;25(3):105–11.
35. Tolksdorf W, Eick C. Rektale, rectal, oral and nasal premedication using midazolam in children aged 1-6 years. A comparative clinical study. Anaesthesist. 1991;40(12):661–7.
36. Roelofse JA, van der Bijl P. Comparison of rectal midazolam and diazepam for premedication in pediatric dental patients. J Oral Maxillofac Surg. 1993;51(5):525–9. https://doi.org/10.1016/s0278-2391(10)80507-5.
37. e Boer AG, Moolenaar F, de Leede LGJ, et al. Rectal drug administration. Clin Pharmacokinet. 1982;7:285–311. https://doi.org/10.2165/00003088-198207040-00002.
38. Lejus C, Renaudin M, Testa S, Malinovsky JM, Vigier T, Souron R. Midazolam for premedication in children: nasal vs. rectal administration. Eur J Anaesthesiol. 1997;14(3):244–9. https://doi.org/10.1046/j.1365-2346.1997.00013.x.

39. Spear RM, Yaster M, Berkowitz ID, Maxwell LG, Bender KS, Naclerio R, Manolio TA, Nichols DG. Preinduction of anesthesia in children with rectally administered midazolam. Anesthesiology. 1991;74(4):670–4. https://doi.org/10.1097/00000542-199104000-00009.
40. Zhang H, Zhang J, Streisand JB. Oral mucosal drug delivery: clinical pharmacokinetics and therapeutic applications. Clin Pharmacokinet. 2002;41(9):661–80. https://doi.org/10.2165/00003088-200241090-00003.
41. Jevon P. Buccolam(®) (buccal midazolam): a review of its use for the treatment of prolonged acute convulsive seizures in the dental practice. Br Dent J. 2012;213(2):81–2. https://doi.org/10.1038/sj.bdj.2012.617.
42. Ashrafi MR, Khosroshahi N, Karimi P, Malamiri RA, Bavarian B, Zarch AV, Mirzaei M, Kompani F. Efficacy and usability of buccal midazolam in controlling acute prolonged convulsive seizures in children. Eur J Paediatr Neurol. 2010;14(5):434–8. https://doi.org/10.1016/j.ejpn.2010.05.009. Epub 2010 Jun 15.
43. Karl HW, Rosenberger JL, Larach MG, et al. Transmucosal administration of midazolam for premedication of pediatric patients. Anesthesiology. 1993;78(5):885–91.
44. Geldner G, Hubmann M, Knoll R, et al. Comparison between three transmucosal routes of administration of midazolam in children. Paediatr Anaesth. 1997;7:103–9.
45. Shanmugaavel AK, Asokan S, John JB, Priya PR, Raaja MT. Comparison of drug acceptance and anxiety between intranasal and sublingual midazolam sedation. Pediatr Dent. 2016;38(2):106–11.
46. Tavassoli-Hojjati S, Mehran M, Haghgoo R, Tohid-Rahbari M, Ahmadi R. Comparison of oral and buccal midazolam for pediatric dental sedation: a randomized, cross-over, clinical trial for efficacy, acceptance and safety. Iran J Pediatr. 2014;24(2):198–206.

Local Anesthetic Techniques in Children

6

6.1 Overview

It has been repeatedly emphasized throughout this book that local anesthesia in conjunction with non-pharmacological behavior guidance techniques is integral for successful outcomes with midazolam. But the administration of local anesthesia in children is a double-edged sword. Its careful and gentle administration will improve child cooperation by enhancing the anxiolytic effect of midazolam. But an unpleasant experience can negatively impact child's behavior possibly leading to an undesired paradoxical reaction. This chapter will streamline a process for the administration of local anesthetic injections in children. It will also describe specific techniques to administer some common intraoral injections like supraperiosteal injections, palatal injections, and the inferior alveolar nerve block with minimal discomfort. Some important clinical considerations related to local anesthesia in children will also be discussed. This will include injection in the maxillary second primary/first permanent molar region, maximum recommended dosage of the anesthetic solution, effectiveness of mandibular molar supraperiosteal injections, and the role of buffering to enhance the effectiveness of the local anesthetic solution.

6.2 Background and Objective

Midazolam possesses antianxiety and sedative properties. It does not possess analgesic properties. It can only alter pain perception and pain reaction by elevating the pain threshold. It does this by creating an environment through its anxiolytic properties, where the child will be indifferent to mild noxious stimuli [1]. But major pain control can be provided only by local anesthesia.

Administration of a local anesthetic injection in a child is a double-edged sword. This is more so in a child under the influence of midazolam. Its administration with minimum discomfort ensures adequate pain control, which may further enhance the

© The Author(s), under exclusive license to Springer Nature Switzerland AG 2024
A. Rao, S. Tiwari, *Midazolam in Pediatric Dentistry*,
https://doi.org/10.1007/978-3-031-45147-8_6

anxiolytic effect of midazolam. But an unpleasant experience during the injection process may lead to negative child behavior. The child displaying negative behavior may try to fight the calming effect of midazolam, possibly leading to an aggressive paradoxical reaction. So administration of local anesthesia with minimum discomfort is an integral part of midazolam sedation.

The ultimate objective of behavior guidance is to deliver pain-free treatment to the child and help the child develop a positive attitude toward dentistry. When the anxious child apprehensively sits or is convinced to sit on the dental chair, the child rightfully expects dental treatment without any discomfort. Adults come to accept some discomfort associated with dental treatment. But we cannot expect young children to experience pain and still cooperate for the treatment. Clinicians treating children are duty-bound to control pain perception, pain reaction, and the actual pain. The combination of midazolam and local anesthesia has the potential to do that.

This chapter will discuss negating the pain associated with the administration of local anesthesia in children through effective skills, attitudes, and techniques by the clinician, ably supported by behavior guidance techniques and moderate sedation with midazolam or inhalation sedation as needed. It will streamline a process consisting of nine steps for the administration of local anesthesia in children. It will also describe specific techniques to administer some common injections with minimal discomfort to children. Detailed descriptions of standard intraoral injection techniques are beyond the scope of the chapter. For details on standard techniques of administering supraperiosteal injections and palatal injections and the various blocks, the reader is referred to other classic, well-established resources on the subject [2, 3].

6.3   The Philosophy of Local Anesthesia in Children

Most adults tolerate the mild pain and discomfort associated with local anesthetic injections to an extent. They are conditioned that an injection will cause a certain amount of discomfort. They would have voluntarily fixed the dental appointment. They will accept the trade-off between the pain caused by the injection and the possible progress and consequences, if the dental disease is neglected, along with the resultant increased expenses.

This is obviously not the case with children. Parents would have brought them to the dental practice fearing progress of the dental disease. Children are not interested in the "dental disease progress-minimal pain of injection trade-off". They view injection as an unnecessary painful experience conditioned from numerous immunization experiences in their childhood [4]. The importance of immunizations is undebatable of course. But, very often, they are administered to an involuntary child under physical restraint with the needle in full view of the child. The unpleasant procedure is quickly completed, and the child is discharged from the practice with verbal reassurances. But Pediatric Dentistry is a different ball game. Here, the local anesthetic injection only marks the beginning of a challenging dental procedure. The child already conditioned to the association of "pain and needles" makes it an even more challenging scenario. It is to the credit of dentists treating children that they routinely provide invasive treatment to children under local anesthesia that would be rarely provided by surgeons in the medical fraternity without general anesthesia [5]. Pediatric Dentists owe this to their training in non-pharmacological behavioral guidance techniques and pharmacological techniques mainly local anesthesia. The addition of moderate sedation to these techniques has further added to the number of apprehensive children where complicated dental treatment has been completed, with all the techniques (*non-pharmacological behavioral guidance, local anesthesia, and moderate sedation*) working in conjunction.

6.4   Are "Painless" Intraoral Injections Possible?

Pain is very subjective. The pain perception and reaction of each child towards intraoral injections can vary depending on various factors like:

- Previous experience with injections
- Subjective fear of injections developed through experiences of other children or adults
- The confidence the child has in the clinician
- Use of effective non-pharmacological techniques by the clinician
- Skill of the clinician administering the injection

The authors will therefore refrain from using the term "painless" local anesthetic techniques. We will rather describe techniques that will realistically aim to administer intraoral injections with "minimal discomfort" to children.

The administration of local anesthesia in children with minimal discomfort should be a conscious effort on the part of the clinician. There is no technique that can ensure it. It is all about following a process and practicing it consistently. New technologies and knowledge will aid and add onto this process making it simpler. There may not be 100% success in this pursuit, because pain perception is subjective more so in children. But, if the clinician follows the process religiously learning through the mistakes along the way, she/he will fulfill the objective of a "minimal discomfort injection" more often than not.

6.5   The Process

To administer intraoral injections with minimal discomfort to children, there lies a process. The process described in this chapter consists of nine steps. The nine steps basically blend the effective use of non-pharmacological behavior guidance techniques with a sound basic intraoral injection technique. The following is a detailed description of the nine steps involved.

6.5.1   Establishing Two-Way Communication

The effective administration of local anesthesia in children requires the imperative use of communicative behavior guidance techniques like tell-show-do, euphemisms, distraction, and verbal positive reinforcements. Establishment of two-way communication is the foundation on which these communicative techniques effectively explain the concept of local anesthesia to the child in an age-appropriate language. In two-way communication, the child proactively responds to the clinician's questions or instructions. For example, when the clinician gives an instruction to the child and asks "have you understood?", the child has to respond with a "Yes" or a "nod" of the head. If the clinician is *not* able to establish two-way communication, then she/he should *not* attempt any treatment especially local anesthesia. Attempting a local anesthetic injection without having established two way communication invariably means heading towards failure.

   Establishing two-way communication with the child is a skill which some clinicians are naturally gifted with. Various aspects of their personality allow them "expressions" or "activities" that gain the child's attention paving the way for two-way communication. But, it is also a skill that can be acquired by the rather introvert clinician, but who is keen to treat children. The clinician with a friendly body language can ask close-ended questions like the child's name and her/his favorite animation character, give the child a choice to pick her/his favorite color, or resort to any other easy conversation, which may encourage the child to respond.

   Establishment of two-way communication is also dependent on the Frankl behavior rating of the child. It is easier to establish communication with the child displaying definitely positive and positive behavior compared to a child displaying negative and definitely negative behavior. Children displaying negative or definitely negative behavior may require anxiolysis and/or the use of non pharmacological techniques like voice modulation to facilitate the establishment of two-way communication. The reader is referred to Chap. 4 for further details on this concept.

   The bottom line is that the first non-negotiable step leading to a successful local anesthetic injection in a child, is the establishment of two-way communication.

6.5.2   Use of Euphemisms

Establishment of two-way communication leads to the effective use of euphemisms. Euphemism is the substitution of a word considered unpleasant or harsh by a pleasant or mild word. In the context of local anesthetic injections in children, the objective of using euphemisms is to create positive images and perceptions about the difficult procedure. Here, it is very important to understand the term "connotations." Connotations are the feelings that a word invokes in an individual. For example, the word "rain" may have positive or negative connotations for different individuals. For some, it may bring in childhood memories of playing and enjoying the rain, but for others, rain may be associated with bad memories like floods, thundering, and various other negative associations. The understanding of "connotations" leads to the effective use of euphemisms.

It is very important to use euphemisms with positive connotations to describe the concept of local anesthesia to children. The authors use the euphemisms "magic water" for the local anesthetic solution and "strong" for the numbness that will set in following the administration of local anesthesia. Children generally have positive connotations about words like "magic" and "strong." So we describe the local anesthetic solution and the soft tissue anesthesia that will set in post the inferior alveolar nerve block as "I will put some *magic water* in your mouth which will make your tooth, lips, cheeks and tongue very *strong*." The resulting positive imagery and perception, helps prepare the child for the process.

But, in spite of the clinician's best efforts, it is inevitable that the child may still feel some discomfort during the local anesthetic process. Here, we can effectively use euphemisms with negative connotations to subtly prepare the child for this possible discomfort. The "enhancing control" [6] technique is first taught to the child. This is a technique where the child assumes an active role in the treatment process by raising her/his hand when she /he feels any discomfort. Now the child is told that "*The bad germs will be running away because of the magic water. But, if they bite, you can let me know by raising your hand*." Words like "bad germs" and "bite" generally have negative connotations. So we try and influence the child's perception by giving an impression that if she/he does feel any discomfort, it is because of the *bite* of the *bad germs*. The doctor is not causing the pain. So if the germs hurt her/him, she/he can raise the hand and inform the doctor, who will give more magic water to chase those bad germs. The child is given an impression that basically the doctor and the child are in one team and they have to fight the germs together.

In summary, euphemisms positive or negative, have to be carefully selected to help the child tide over the challenging local anesthetic process.

6.5.3 Instructions to the Parents

Parental presence or absence in the operatory has always been an ongoing debate in Pediatric Dentistry. There are advantages and advocates to both parental presence and absence [7]. The current general consensus is that parents prefer to be present with their child inside the operatory during dental treatment [8]. The authors also prefer the presence of parents in the operatory during the treatment. In addition to all the advantages of parental presence cited [7], the parents also get to appreciate firsthand, the challenges of child management and the effort put in by the clinician towards scaling those challenges. The authors in fact routinely encourage one parent of young children to be in their close proximity and contact on the dental chair, during the initial appointments (Fig. 6.1).

The child's feet resting on the parent's lap provides emotional security for both the child and the parent. The parents though need to be given clear instructions upfront by the front desk against sidestepping the clinician's authority inside the operatory. This is especially critical during the process of the local

Fig. 6.1 Parent in proximity of the child on the dental chair

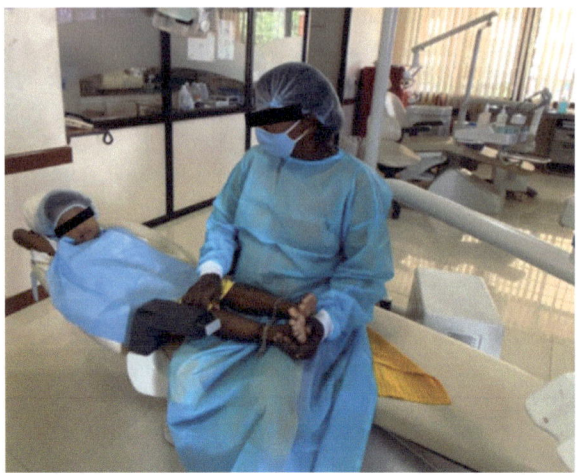

anesthetic injection, when the clinician is making an effort to keep the syringe below the child's line of sight while taking it towards the oral cavity. The parent may with all the good intentions ask the child to close her/his eyes or gently clutch the child's hands or feet, alerting the child's suspicions to something unpleasant.

The parents should be reassured at the front desk that the child is in very good, trained, and experienced hands. It should be reinforced that their presence in the operatory should be passive and only to the extent of providing emotional support to their child. Once the local anesthetic injection is successfully administered, the parents are very often amazed at the expertise with which the difficult procedure was completed. This leads to them developing trust and respect for the clinician and many parents voluntarily opt to stay out of the operatory for the future appointments.

6.5.4 Applying the Topical Anesthetic

Very often, the effectiveness of the topical anesthetic is compromised due to an incorrect protocol. The topical anesthetic applied with the correct technique partially anesthetizes the mucosa to a 2–3 mm depth aiding in an atraumatic penetration of the needle into the mucosa. The site of injection should be dried and cleaned with gauze, and a small amount of flavored topical anesthetic should be applied with a sterile cotton applicator tip. It should be left in contact with the tissues for at least 2 minutes, though the time can vary between various topical anesthetic drugs. For 5% lidocaine, the onset time to surface anesthesia is approximately 2–5 minutes, whereas for 20% benzocaine, it is said to be 30 seconds [9]. "Tooth jam" and "toothpaste" are good euphemisms in the authors' experience to introduce the topical anesthetic gel to the child.

6.5.5 Needle Selection and Assembling the Syringe

There is a lot of discussion on the ideal choice of the length and gauge of the needle for administering local anesthetic injections. For young children, the authors prefer an ultrashort 30 gauge needle for buccal supraperiosteal injections, palatal injections and for the first stage of the modified two-stage inferior alveolar nerve block (IANB) technique (*explained later*). In these injections, the aspiration risks are minimal. Aspiration is an important consideration when selecting the 30 gauge needle because of the ambiguity in studies reporting the ability of higher gauge needles to reliably aspirate blood [10, 11].

> Gauge of the needle refers to the internal diameter of the needle hole. The higher the gauge, the smaller the diameter.

Even assuming that blood may be aspirated through the higher gauge needles like the 30 gauge needle, the pressure required for the aspiration purpose may disengage the harpoon from the rubber plunger [12]. For the second stage of the IANB (*explained later*) where the needle will be penetrated deep towards the bone in a vascular-rich area, the authors prefer a 25 or 27 gauge short needle, which will aspirate more reliably.

When the topical anesthesia is taking effect, the assembling of the syringe should be completed by the assistant behind or out of sight of the child. Once the cartridge is mounted into the syringe, the assistant should expel a few drops to check the free flow of the solution. She/he then passes the uncapped syringe behind the child's head to the clinician.

6.5.6 Keeping the Syringe Out of the Child's Line of Sight

The clinician receives the uncapped syringe from the assistant and brings the syringe under the child's chin into the mouth (Fig. 6.2).

An audiovisual device mounted on the ceiling, above the dental chair, is an effective distraction during this process (See Sect. 6.5.9).

The blinding of the child to the syringe and needle is very important because there is no good reason for the child to see the needle or the syringe. There will already be an established fear of needles fueled objectively and subjectively in most children. Once the child sees the syringe with the needle, no amount of rationalization will likely convince the child about accepting the injection.

But what does the clinician do if the child does see the uncapped syringe? Well, it is an uphill task from there. The most important *"don't"* here is that the clinician should never try to hide or conceal the syringe. In fact, she/he should calmly but quickly expel a few drops on the child's hand and reinforce the earlier

Fig. 6.2 The syringe out
of the child's line of sight

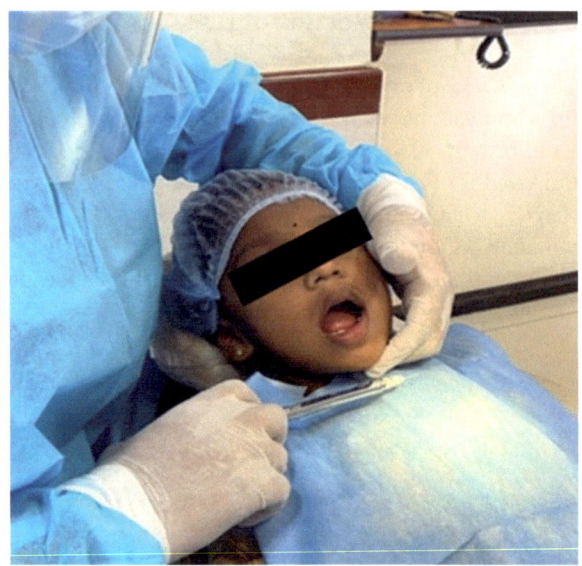

described euphemism of "magic water." If the needle is an ultrashort 30 gauge type, the child may not feel threatened and may ease back into the audiovisual distraction.

6.5.7 Needle Insertion

The following is an effective and well-known technique that aids atraumatic needle insertions into the mucosa.

The tissue at the site of needle insertion is stretched and made taut. This helps the sharp stainless steel needle (bevel facing bone) penetrate the tissue with minimum resistance compared to penetrating loose tissue. The stretched taut tissue is pulled over the needle. This stretch and manipulation of the mucosa is supposed to lessen the pain associated with the needle penetration according to gate's control theory of pain. The stretch and the mucosal manipulation activates more large nerve fibers associated with touch and inhibits the small fibers associated with pain [13, 14]. A distractive environment to the needle insertion can also be created by the external application of commercially available dental vibratory devices. These devices can further be coupled with a cold gel (Fig. 6.3).

Their application is based on the theory that they cause the brain cells to relay the non-pain signals such as vibration or cold, masking the pain signals triggered by the injection [15–17].

Fig. 6.3 Dental vibratory device, Buzzy®, MMJ Labs, Atlanta GA, USA

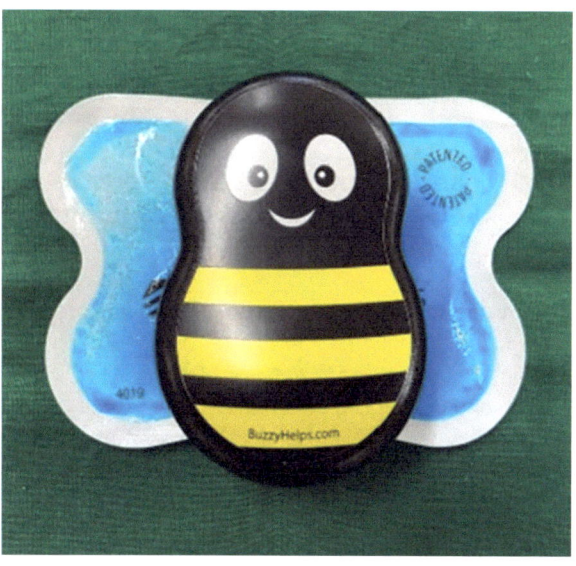

6.5.8   Slow Deposition of the Local Anesthetic Solution

There are two points in the process of the local anesthetic injection that can cause pain. The first is during needle insertion into the tissues, which was discussed in the above paragraph. The second is from the pressure and soft tissue expansion due to the initial deposition of the solution into the mucosa. To negate this pain, it is emphasized that the initial deposition of the local anesthetic solution into the tissues should always be in drops and never in a flow. The deposition of the first few drops is especially very critical. The first drop expelled should be of the smallest volume possible by pushing the plunger or the thumb ring of the syringe. This is subjective and will depend on the dexterity and skill of the operator and improves with practice. After a delay of a couple of seconds, the second small drop is deposited and so on with the needle also being simultaneously pushed deeper into the mucosa. The volume of the solution expelled can gradually increase following the initial few drops. A slow injection involves the deposition of 1 mL of the local anesthetic solution in not less than a minute [18].

The computer-controlled local anesthetic delivery (CCLAD) system can be a very useful alternative to the dexterity and skill required to deposit the local anesthetic solution in controlled volumes and pressure. They deliver the solution at a preprogrammed rate of flow and pressure. In addition, the handpiece held with a pen grasp results in improved ergonomics and tactile sensation for the clinician. Its non-threatening appearance also helps a great deal with children. The Wand STA® (Milestone Scientific, Livingston, NJ), Comfort Control Syringe (CCS; Dentsply, USA), QuickSleeper (Dentalhitec, France), and Dentapen (Juvaplus SA, Neuchatel,

Switzerland) are some of the popular CCLAD systems available commercially [19]. The CCLAD systems have also proven to be very effective in delivering periodontal ligament injections in children [20].

6.5.9 Use of Distraction, Verbal Positive/Negative Reinforcement, and Voice Modulation During the Injection Process

Post insertion of the needle, during the slow expression of the local anesthetic solution, a ceiling-mounted audiovisual distraction above the dental chair playing animations, could be a very useful distraction (Fig. 6.4). The clinician could also opt for any other suitable distraction.

The clinician should also positively reinforce the desired behavior by generously praising the child continuously as a "brave girl/boy," "excellent," and "I am proud of you." Negative reinforcement can also effectively be used as a distraction by telling the child that the process will be over at the slow count by the operator to the number 20. The tone of the clinician should be monotonous and soothing.

But, sometimes, a slight discomfort may prompt the child to pull the clinician's hand. At this point, the clinician should tactfully use voice modulation. Parent consent for voice modulation should already have been obtained before the local anesthetic injection in anticipation. The change from the monotone to a sudden and short *"DO NOT DO THAT"* very effectively surprises the child who will likely revert her/

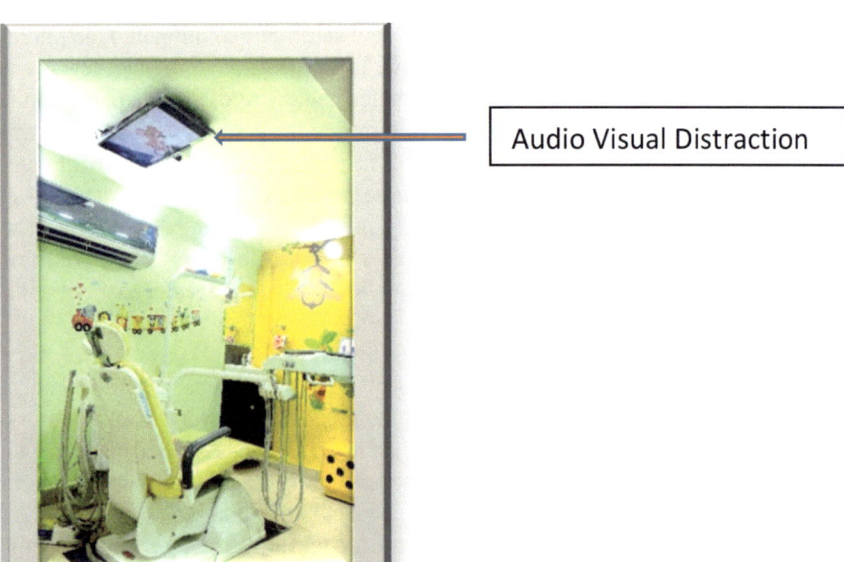

Audio Visual Distraction

Fig. 6.4 Audiovisual distraction on the ceiling above the dental chair

his action. This should immediately be rewarded by the clinician with generous praise in a soothing tone boosting the child's self-esteem.

After the completion of the injection process, the clinician brings the syringe out of the mouth, under the child's chin, and passes it to the assistant out of the child's line of sight. The child is again reminded of the "magic" that will start around the mouth and warned not to chew on the lips, cheeks, or tongue. When the soft tissue anesthesia sets in, the child can be given a hand mirror to reassure the child that her/his face still looks the same and the "magic" will disappear in a few hours. The introduction of the "soft tissue anesthesia" reversal agent phentolamine mesylate has significantly reduced the duration of residual soft tissue anesthesia and the consequent soft tissue trauma in children [19].

The authors at the end of the nine-step description want to emphasize that local anesthesia in children is a phase in the overall treatment process. It requires dedicated time, and the above described process has to be meticulously followed for successful administrations of local anesthesia in children.

6.6 Local Anesthetic Techniques in Children

With the background knowledge of the nine steps required for the administration of injections in children, we will now describe specific techniques for three commonly used injections in children:

– Buccal/labial supraperiosteal injection
– Inferior alveolar nerve block
– Palatal injections

The authors believe that, with sufficient practice, the clinician practicing these techniques will consistently be able to attain her/his objective of delivering intraoral injections in children with minimal discomfort. The techniques described are to be used in conjunction with the preceding nine steps.

6.6.1 The Buccal/Labial Supraperiosteal Injection

6.6.1.1 Difference Between a Supraperiosteal Injection and an Infiltration

In a supraperiosteal injection, as the name suggests, the local anesthetic solution is deposited on the periosteum near the apex of the tooth. Hence, the syringe should also be directed at an angle such that the needle tip is on the periosteum near the apex of the tooth (Fig. 6.5).

Infiltration is the incorrect term that only indicates the injection of the local anesthetic solution directly into the tissues of the tooth to be treated.

Fig. 6.5 Angled syringe for the supraperiosteal injection

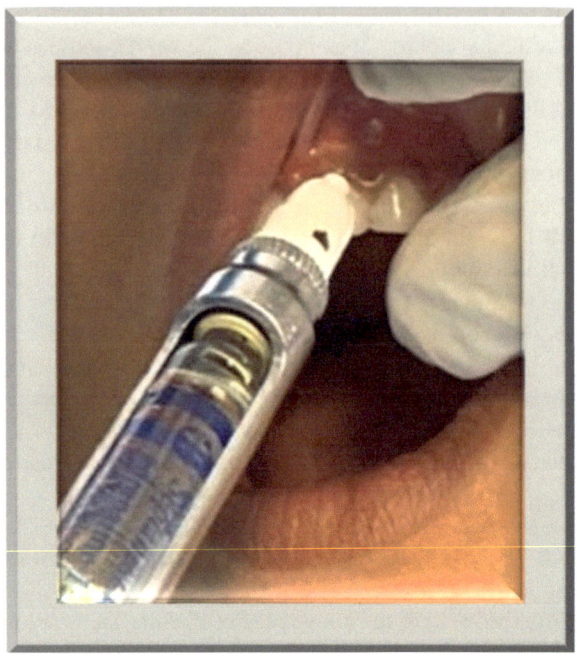

6.6.1.2 Shorter Syringes for Children

Ideally, syringes designed for intraoral injections in children should be smaller/shorter than conventional syringes. It is ergonomically difficult to use a long syringe in the small oral cavity of the child. Since shorter syringes are not currently available commercially, we have to *relatively* shorten the length of the conventional syringe. We can do this by (Fig. 6.6):

- **Emptying almost two-thirds of the cartridge and retaining only about 0.8 mL of the local anesthetic solution**
- The rationale here is twofold. The first is that 0.8 mL volume is sufficient for supraperiosteal injections in children. The second is that emptying almost two-thirds of the cartridge brings the thumb inside the thumb ring being closer to the finger grip. This affords much greater control to the operator in expressing small volumes of the local anesthetic solution. It also enables the operator to use a finger rest on the child's face, which helps stabilize the syringe during needle insertion (Fig. 6.7).
- **Using the ultrashort 30 gauge needle**
- The ultrashort needle suffices for supraperiosteal injections in children for most situations. The use of the ultrashort needle not only causes less needle deflection inside the tissues but also further decreases the overall length of the syringe.

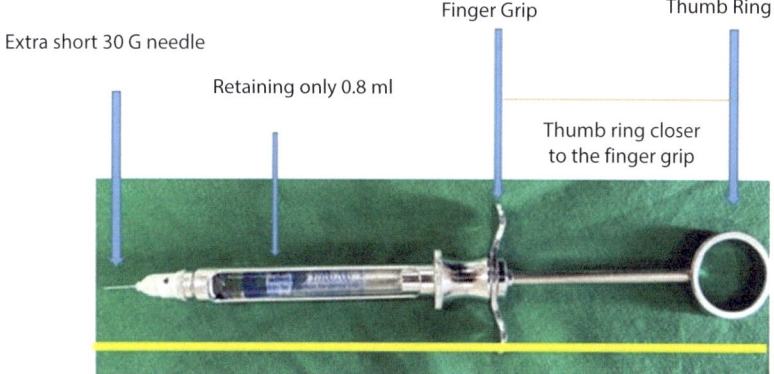

Finger Grip   Thumb Ring

Extra short 30 G needle

Retaining only 0.8 ml

Thumb ring closer
to the finger grip

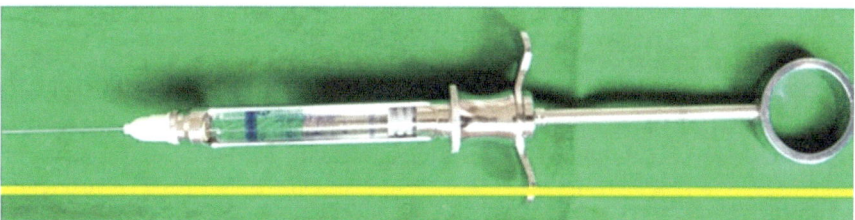

Fig. 6.6 Making the syringe relatively shorter

Fig. 6.7 Finger rest
facilitated by the shorter
syringe

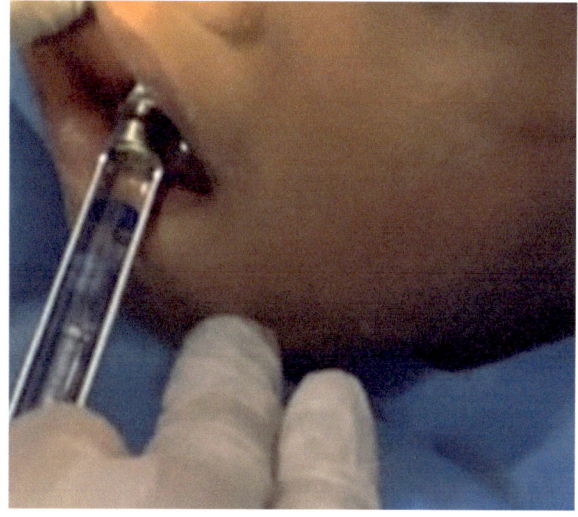

6.6.1.3 The Supraperiosteal Injection Technique

The buccal/labial mucosa is made taut and stretched over the needle so that it penetrates 2 mm into the mucosa (Sects. 6.5.7 and 6.5.8). A drop of the local anesthetic solution is deposited. The first drop expelled should be of the smallest volume possible. This is subjective and will depend on the dexterity and skill of the operator and improves with practice. After a couple of seconds, the needle is advanced an mm further into the mucosa and another drop is deposited. This cycle of injecting small drops at 2-second intervals is continued till the needle is about 3–5 mm into the mucosa on the periosteum near the vicinity of the tooth apex. At this level, about 0.6 mL of the solution is deposited slowly following aspiration. The process is completed in a minute, and the total amount of local anesthetic solution deposited should be approximately 0.8 mL.

6.6.2   Palatal Anesthesia with the Intra-papillary Technique [21]

This technique is applicable to both anterior and posterior teeth. The buccal/labial periosteal injection is administered as described. A fresh cartridge is loaded, and again only 0.8 mL of the solution is retained to aid better control. Once labial/buccal soft tissue anesthesia is confirmed, the syringe with the ultrashort 30 gauge needle is reinserted 1 mm into the base of the buccal/labial papilla causing blanching (Fig. 6.8).

   A drop of the solution is deposited, and the needle progresses towards the palatal tissues simultaneously depositing the solution in drops. The key here is that the

Fig. 6.8 Needle inserted into the base of the labial papilla

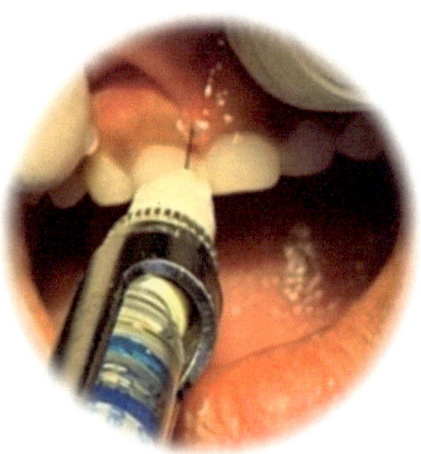

drops should be deposited under moderate pressure. The objective should be to blanch the opposing palatal tissue as blanching is also a sign of anesthesia.

If moderate pressure sufficient to blanch the opposing palatal papilla is not generated, then the clinician should withdraw the needle slightly and redirect it more apically toward the palatal alveolar crest. The drops should *not be* deposited without pressure as the solution will leak and flow into the oral cavity resulting in a bitter taste. It should also be noted that the objective is to blanch the palatal papilla and the tissues in close vicinity. The needle should not penetrate through the palatal papilla. Once a few drops are deposited under moderate pressure blanching the palatal papilla, the syringe is withdrawn completely. The palatal anesthesia is now further reinforced by injecting a couple of drops directly into the palatal papilla. If it is a posterior tooth, the process is followed both in the mesial and the distal papilla. The anesthesia developed through this procedure will be sufficient for restorative procedures like preformed metal crowns or application of the rubber dam clamp. The same procedure can be replicated if mandibular lingual anesthesia is desired.

If more profound palatal anesthesia is required as for an extraction, the anesthesia needs to be reinforced further. The cotton applicator tip used to apply the topical anesthetic is pressed against the palatal tissue near the approximate root apex till blanching appears. The anesthesia is now reinforced by injecting slowly just above the cotton applicator tip (Fig. 6.9).

This intra-papillary technique of obtaining palatal anesthesia can also be carried out with a 1 mL disposable insulin syringe with an ultrashort 8 mm, 30 gauge needle (Fig. 6.10).

Fig. 6.9 Procedure for profound palatal anesthesia

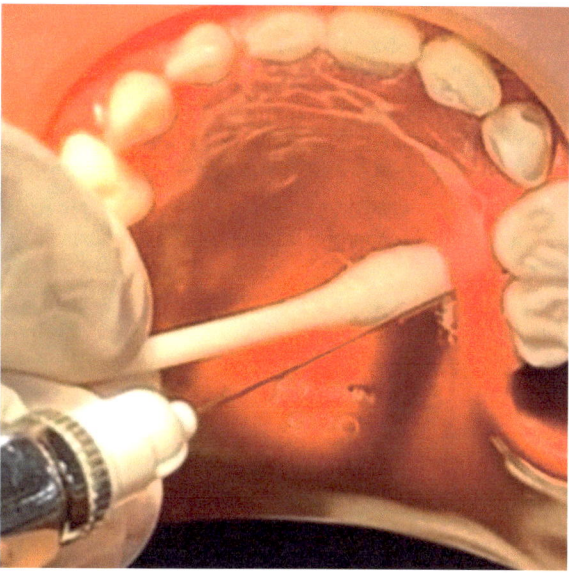

Fig. 6.10 The disposable
insulin syringe

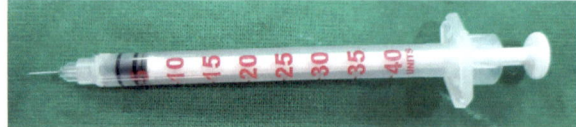

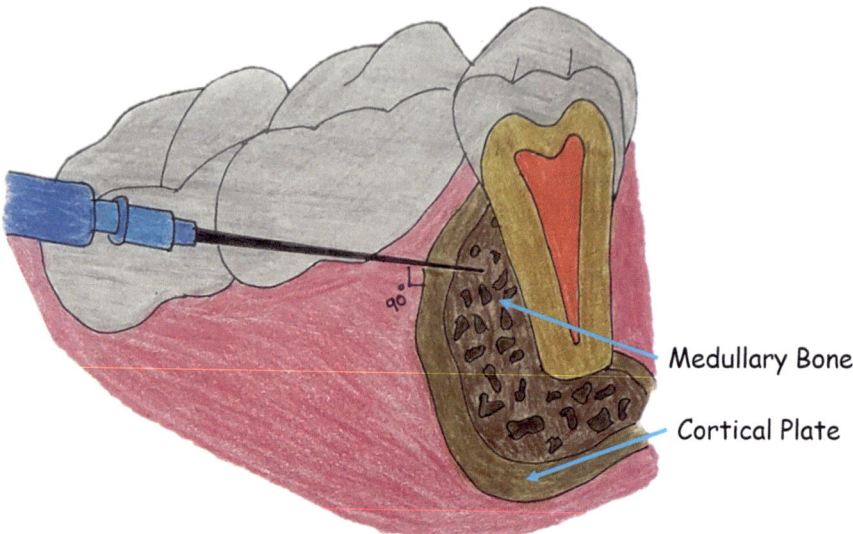

Medullary Bone

Cortical Plate

Fig. 6.11 Intraseptal injection

A distinction has to be made between the intra-papillary and intraseptal injections. The intraseptal injection is almost similar in technique to the intra-papillary injection. But post anesthetizing the labial/buccal soft tissues, the needle is inserted into the intraseptal bone. The distal intraseptal bone of the tooth to be anesthetized is utilized for a posterior tooth. About 0.2 mL of the anesthetic solution should be deposited under resistance. The decreased bone density in children allows its use as a supplemental technique to aid pulpal anesthesia (Fig. 6.11).

There have also been reports of the ability of 4% articaine to diffuse through the hard and soft tissues from buccal infiltrations to anesthetize the palatal and lingual tissues. But results in children have not been consistent to recommend the practice clinically [22].

6.6.3 The Modified Two-Stage Inferior Alveolar Nerve Block (IANB) Technique

Before we deal with the modified two-stage IANB, let us first understand the conventional two-stage IANB. It is one of the techniques explained in literature to administer an IANB with minimal discomfort [23]. The technique is as follows.

6.6.3.1 The Conventional Two-Stage IANB

The IANB here is administered in two stages. The first stage involves administration of a small volume of the local anesthetic solution under the mucosal surface. A 27 gauge, 1 inch needle is penetrated 2 mm into the mucosa, and a drop of the local anesthetic solution is deposited. After a couple of seconds, the needle is advanced an mm further into the mucosa, and another drop is deposited. This cycle of injecting small drops at 2-second intervals is continued till the needle is about 6–8 mm into the mucosa. At this level into the mucosa, about 0.3 mL of the solution is deposited gently. The first stage is completed in a minute, and the total amount of local anesthetic solution deposited will be 0.5 mL. In the second stage performed 5 minutes later, the needle is reinserted into the pre-anesthetized mucosa and advanced slowly to contact the medial aspect of the mandibular ramus. 1 mL of the local anesthetic solution is slowly deposited in the area over a minute following negative aspiration. A total of 1.5 mL of the local anesthetic solution will be deposited at the end of the two stages [24].

The rationale of the technique is that, with the mucosa pre-anesthetized in the first stage, the clinician, in the second stage, can focus on contacting the bone on the medial aspect of the mandibular ramus as close to the inferior alveolar canal as possible. The clinician does not have to simultaneously deal with the dual challenge of potential pain during needle insertion/progress and contacting the bone at adequate depth.

6.6.3.2 The Modified Two-Stage IANB

The drawback of the conventional two-stage technique in children is the potential for pain during needle insertion and deposition of the local anesthetic solution in the first stage. A modification to the two-stage technique uses two separate cartridges and two different needles for the two stages of the IANB to negate the drawbacks of the conventional technique as described below.

The First Stage of the Modified Two-Stage IANB

In the first stage, an ultrashort, 10 mm, 30 gauge needle is used along with a cartridge containing only about 0.5 mL of the local anesthetic solution. The ultrashort needle results in less deflection [24], and the fine 30 gauge needle imperceptibly penetrates the mucosa (Please refer to Sect. 6.5.7). Studies have reported no difference in pain perception by the patients injected with 25, 27, or 30 gauge needles [25]. But these studies have been validated only on adults. There is a need for further research in this area among children. In a study on children, Ram D and coauthors reported that children cried less during the mandibular block administered with a 30 gauge needle compared to a 27 gauge needle [26]. The rationale to emptying the cartridge retaining only 0.5 mL of the solution as explained in Sect. 6.5.8 is to aid better control towards expelling the smallest volumes for the first few drops of the injection by bringing the thumb ring closer to the finger grip of the syringe. It also enables the operator to use a finger rest on the child's face, which helps stabilize the syringe during needle insertion.

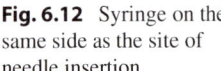 **Fig. 6.12** Syringe on the same side as the site of needle insertion

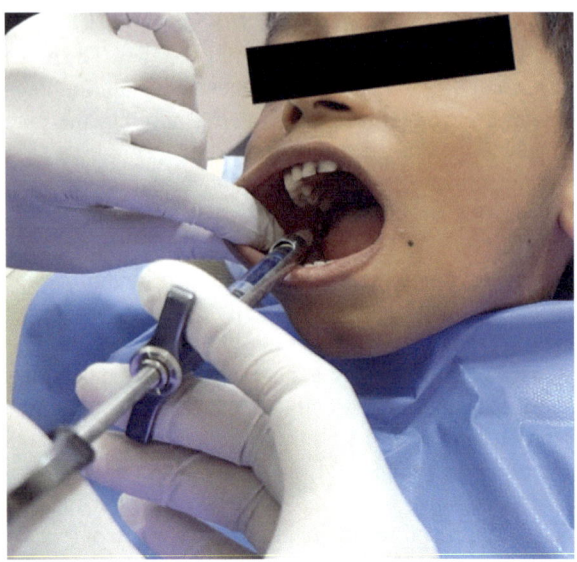

The syringe in the first stage is positioned on the same side as the site of needle insertion (Fig. 6.12).

In the traditional IANB technique, the needle and syringe approach the site of needle insertion from the opposite side. But the tongue in young children can involuntarily push against the barrel of the syringe in this approach. Hence, in the first stage of the modified two-stage IANB, it is recommended that the syringe approaches the site of needle insertion from the same side. Positioning the syringe on the same side as the site of needle insertion gives more control to the clinician by negating the potential interference by the tongue [27]. The buccal mucosa is made taut and stretched over the needle, so that it penetrates 2 mm into the mucosa. A drop of the local anesthetic solution is deposited. The first drop expelled should be of smallest volume possible by pushing the plunger (thumb ring of the syringe). This is subjective and will depend on the dexterity and skill of the operator and improves with practice. After a couple of seconds, the needle is advanced an mm further into the mucosa, and another drop is deposited. This cycle of injecting small drops at 2-s intervals is continued till the needle is about 6–8 mm into the mucosa. At this level into the mucosa, about 0.3 mL of the solution is deposited slowly following aspiration. The first stage is completed in a minute, and the total amount of local anesthetic solution deposited will be 0.5 mL.

A 1 mL disposable insulin syringe with an ultrashort 8 mm, 30 gauge needle can alternatively be used in the first stage [13, 24, 27]. The 1 mL of the insulin syringe is marked by 40 units on the barrel (Fig. 6.13).

The 40 units is indicated by graduations where the interval between 2 graduations represent 1 unit (Fig. 6.14).

Fig. 6.13 1 mL on the syringe marked by 40 units

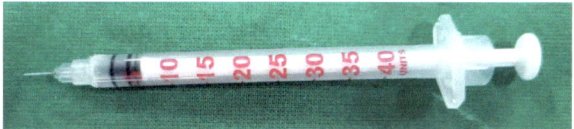

The rationale of using the insulin syringe for the first stage is that the small diameter of the barrel and plunger can hypothetically lead to the release of smaller drops of local anesthetic solution when the plunger is pushed by 0.5 units [24]. Smaller drops lead to less expansion and less discomfort during the deposition of the local anesthetic solution in the first stage.

The Second Stage of the Modified Two-Stage IANB

The second stage is performed 5 minutes later with a new cartridge and a new 27 gauge needle assembled into the syringe. The 27 gauge needle is used in the second stage as the area near the inferior alveolar foramen is a vascular-rich area, hence requiring reliable aspiration. The needle is inserted into the pre-anesthetized mucosa and advanced slowly to contact the medial aspect of the mandibular ramus. 1 mL of the local anesthetic solution is slowly deposited in the area over a minute, following negative aspiration. A total of 1.5 mL of the local anesthetic solution will be deposited at the end of the two stages.

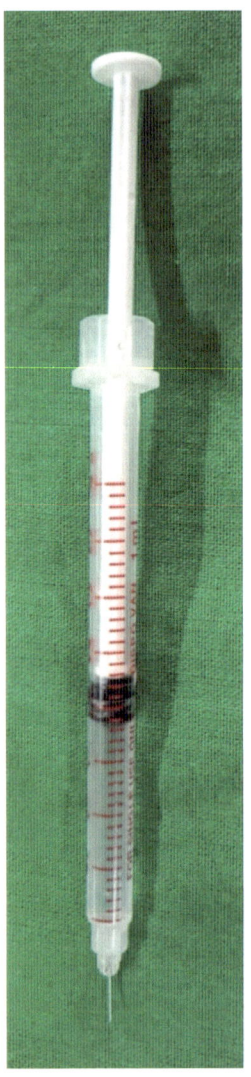

Fig. 6.14 The 40 units on the insulin syringe indicated by graduations

6.7   Additional Considerations for Local Anesthesia in Children

6.7.1   Injection in the Maxillary Second Primary/First Permanent Molar Region

The zygomatic process of the maxilla can often be a hindrance for the supraperiosteal injection in the maxillary first permanent molar and the maxillary second primary molar region. A single supraperiosteal injection between the buccal roots of the molar *may not* result in profound anesthesia for restorative or pulpal procedures. The posterior and middle superior alveolar nerve need to be anesthetized separately. Buccal supraperiosteal injections mesial and distal to the respective mesial and distal roots of the tooth should solve this clinical problem.

If the maxillary primary molar remains sensitive even after the administration of the two supraperiosteal injections, then accessory innervation should be suspected from the palatal nerves, due to the widely flared palatal root of the maxillary primary molar [28] (Fig. 6.15). Administration of palatal anesthesia should solve this clinical problem.

Fig. 6.15 Widely flared palatal root of the maxillary primary second molar

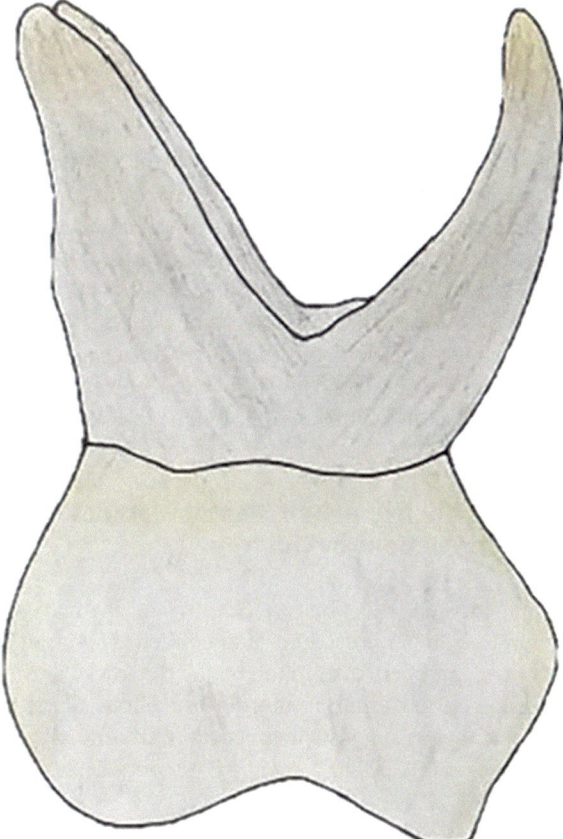

6.7.2   Maximum Recommended Dosage (MRD)

Midazolam and local anesthetic solutions are both central nervous system depressants, and the actions are synergistic. It is very important for the clinician to understand that violating maximum recommended dosages for either drug could lead to complications. In the event of a complication, management further becomes challenging because the clinical presentations of overdosing could be similar for both drugs (e.g., loss of consciousness). Hence, it is prudent to respect dosing regimens of the individual drugs.

In the case of local anesthesia in children, there are well-established definite ground rules to prevent overdosing. These include:

– Customizing the MRD for each individual child, based on the recommended dosage for the specific local anesthetic drug
– Performing multiple aspirations in various planes, which not only prevents inadvertent intravascular injections but also slows the speed of drug administration
– Use of 25 or 27 gauge needles for nerve block injections for reliable aspirations

6.7.2.1   Calculation of MRD

Let us take the example of 2% lidocaine with 1:100,000 epinephrine to understand the calculation of MRD in children. The MRD for 2% lidocaine with 1:100,000 epinephrine is 7.0 mg/kg body weight [4]. Assuming the child's weight to be 14 kg, the MRD is calculated as $7 \times 14 = 98$ mg.

2% translates to 20 mg/mL of the local anesthetic drug. That means 1 mL of the solution contains 20 mg of the drug. Hence, 98 mg will be contained in 4.9 mL of the local anesthetic solution. Hence, the clinician should be very conscious *not* to administer more than 4.9 mL of the drug in one appointment.

Similar calculations can be performed for 4% articaine with 1:100,000 adrenaline, which is the other popular local anesthetic drug in Pediatric Dentistry. The MRD for this drug is 7.0 mg/kg body weight.

With regard to overdosage, articaine with an elimination half-life of 27 minutes (it is eliminated from the blood in 162 minutes or six half-lives) [19], along with its increased rate of success in infiltrations, makes it a preferred local anesthetic in children.

6.7.3   Effectiveness of Mandibular Molar Supraperiosteal Injections in Children

Supraperiosteal injections are effective till the mandibular first primary molars for restorative/pulpal procedures and extraction. But, in the region of the second primary and first permanent molars, the thickness of the cortical plate precludes the diffusion of the solution into the cancellous bone, making it less effective. But recent evidence suggests that buccal infiltration of articaine is a viable alternative to IANB with lignocaine in pediatric patients for treating mandibular molars [29]. 4% articaine with 1:100,000 adrenaline has also shown to be superior to 2% lidocaine with 1:100,000 adrenaline in anesthetizing teeth requiring root canal treatment with irreversible pulpitis via the inferior alveolar nerve block [30]. This is a recommendation for adults though, and more research in this area is required in children. But the authors still recommend the inferior alveolar nerve block for pulpal or surgical procedures in the region of the mandibular second primary and the first permanent molars. This recommendation holds good regardless of the drug used, be it 2% lidocaine or 4% articaine [31]. The effectiveness can be further increased by buffering the local anesthetic solution (*see below*) and working in conjunction with inhalation sedation. The block can be supplemented with buffered articaine infiltration or intraseptal injection as necessary, keeping the MRD in mind.

6.7.4 Buffering the Local Anesthetic Solution [32, 33]

6.7.4.1 The Rationale of Buffering
The addition of adrenaline and the antioxidant sodium bisulfite to local anesthetic solutions, decreases the pH of the solution to 3.5. At this acidic pH, almost the entire percentage of the molecules in the local anesthetic solution are in an ionized or inactive form. This low pH can also cause a burning sensation during its administration. Once injected, the body naturally buffers the anesthetic solution to the body pH of 7.4. At this pH, the percentage of the molecules in the local anesthetic solution in a deionized or active form increase considerably. The deionized molecule form is lipid-soluble. This allows it to diffuse into the lipid-rich nerve membrane, into the nerve and the sodium channels inside, thereby blocking nerve conduction and clinically producing the effect of local anesthesia. But the natural buffering process is slow, delaying the onset of anesthesia. Now, if the pH of the local anesthetic solution could be increased to 7.4 before injecting it into the tissues, a large percentage of molecules in the local anesthetic solution will be already in an active form. This will potentially have three advantages:

1. Lack of burning sensation during the injection process.
2. Quick onset of action due to a large percentage of solution already in an active form.
3. A 6000-fold increase in the number of active molecules, which can theoretically provide a more profound anesthetic effect. This may especially be clinically useful in cases of irreversible pulpitis.

6.7.4.2 The Buffering Process
This increase in pH of the local anesthetic solution prior to the injection can be brought about by the addition of 8.4% sodium bicarbonate solution, which is

commonly used to manage acidosis associated with medical conditions. Sodium bicarbonate is added to the local anesthetic solution with adrenaline in the ratio of 10:1 [34]. For a 1.7 mL cartridge, 0.17 mL sodium bicarbonate is added after dispelling an equivalent volume of the local anesthetic solution from the cartridge. It has to be done immediately before the injection because the local anesthetic solution containing sodium bicarbonate has a limited shelf life. Immediately injecting the buffered solution (within 30–45 seconds) also preserves free carbon dioxide (CO_2), which is said to considerably enhance the potency of the local anesthetic solution [35]. Automated buffering systems are also available, which make the buffering process more precise and convenient, to inject the solution immediately after buffering [19].

Clinically Relevant Points

1. Administration of local anesthesia with minimum discomfort ensures adequate pain control, which may further enhance the anxiolytic effect of midazolam. But an unpleasant experience during the injection process may lead to negative child behavior and an undesired paradoxical reaction.

2. Clinicians treating children are duty-bound to control pain perception, pain reaction, and the actual pain. The combination of midazolam and local anesthesia precisely does that.

3. Administration of local anesthetic injections in children is a process that involves nine steps. They are:
   (a) Establishing two-way communication
   (b) Use of euphemisms
   (c) Instructions to the parents
   (d) Topical anesthesia
   (e) Needle selection and assembling the syringe
   (f) Keeping the syringe out of the child's line of sight
   (g) Needle insertion
   (h) Slow deposition of the local anesthetic solution
   (i) Use of distraction, verbal positive and negative reinforcement, and voice control

4. Syringes in children need to be smaller to aid better control during the injection process. The length of the syringe for supraperiosteal injections can be reduced relatively by emptying the cartridge and retaining only about 0.8 mL of the local anesthetic solution and by the use of an ultra-short 30 gauge needle.

5. The intra-papillary technique is an effective way of administering palatal injections.

6. The modified two-stage technique is an effective technique of administering the IANB in children.

7. A single supraperiosteal injection between the buccal roots of the molar <u>may not</u> result in profound anesthesia for restorative or pulpal procedures in the maxillary second primary/first permanent molar region. The posterior and middle superior alveolar nerve and the palatal nerves may need to be anesthetized separately.

8. Midazolam and local anesthesia are both central nervous system depressants, and the actions are synergistic. It is very important for the clinician to understand that violating maximum recommended dosages for either drug could lead to complications.

9. On current evidence, the inferior alveolar nerve block may still be the injection of choice for pulpal or surgical procedures in the region of the mandibular second primary and the first permanent molars.

10. Buffering the local anesthetic solution may have three advantages:
    (a) Lack of burning sensation during the injection process
    (b) Quick onset of action due to a large percentage of solution already in an active form
    (c) A 6000-fold increase in the number of active molecules, which can theoretically provide a more profound anesthetic effect

References

1. Becker DE, Bennett CR. Intravenous and intramuscular sedation. In: Dionne RA, Phero JC, Becker DE, editors. Management of pain and anxiety in the dental office. 1st ed. WE Saunders Company; 2002. p. 235–60.
2. Malamed SF. Techniques of maxillary anesthesia. In: Handbook of local anesthesia. 7th ed. St. Louis, MO: Elsevier; 2020. p. 204–38.
3. Malamed SF. Techniques of mandibular anesthesia. In: Handbook of local anesthesia. 7th ed. St. Louis, MO: Elsevier; 2020. p. 239–67.
4. Schwartz S, Kupietzky A. Local anesthesia. In: Wright GZ, Kupietzky A, editors. Behavior management in dentistry for children. 2nd ed. Wiley Blackwell; 2014. p. 107–24.
5. Ganzberg SI. Deep sedation and GA. In: Wilson S, editor. Oral sedation for dental procedures in children. Berlin: Springer; 2015. p. 157–71.
6. American Academy of Pediatric Dentistry. Behavior guidance for the pediatric dental patient. The reference manual of pediatric dentistry. Chicago, IL: American Academy of Pediatric Dentistry; 2020. p. 292–310.
7. Shellar B. Influence of the family. In: Wright GZ, Kupietzky A, editors. Behavior management in dentistry for children. 2nd ed. Wiley Blackwell; 2014. p. 35–52.
8. Shroff S, Hughes C, Mobley C. Attitudes and preferences of parents about being present in the dental operatory. Pediatr Dent 2015;37(1):51–5.
9. Aghababaie ST, Monteiro J, Stratigaki E, Ashley PF. Techniques for effective local anaesthetic administration for the paediatric patient. Br Dent J. 2020;229(12):779–85. https://doi.org/10.1038/s41415-020-2453-2.

10. Foldes FF, McNall PG. Toxicity of local anesthetics in man. Dent Clin N Am. 1961;5:257–8.
11. Trapp LD, Davies RO. Aspiration as a function of hypodermic needle internal diameter in the in-vivo human upper limb. Anesth Prog. 1980;27(2):49–51.
12. Malamed SF. The needle. In: Handbook of local anesthesia. 7th ed. St. Louis, MO: Elsevier; 2020. p. 99–110.
13. Rao A, Thakkar D, Rao A, Karuna YM, Srikant N. Evaluation of a modified two-stage inferior alveolar nerve block technique: a preliminary investigation. Dent Hypotheses. 2017;8:34.
14. Wilson S. Non pharmacologic issues in pain perception and control. In: Pinkham JR, Casamassimo PS, Fields HW, McTigue DJ, Nowak A, editors. Pediatric dentistry—infancy through adolescence. 4th ed. St. Louis, MO: Saunders, An imprint of Elsevier; 2005. p. 96–107.
15. Canbulat N, Ayhan F, Inal S. Effectiveness of external cold and vibration for procedural pain relief during peripheral intravenous cannulation in pediatric patients. Pain Manag Nurs. 2015;16(1):33–9.
16. Kearl YL, Yanger S, Montero S, Morelos-Howard E, Claudius I. Does combined use of the J-tip® and buzzy® device decrease the pain of venipuncture in a pediatric population? J Pediatr Nurs. 2015;30(6):829–33.
17. Şahiner NC, Inal S, Akbay AS. The effect of combined stimulation of external cold and vibration during immunization on pain and anxiety levels in children. J Perianesth Nurs. 2015;30(3):228–35.
18. Malamed SF. Basic injection technique. 7th ed. St. Louis, MO: Elsevier; 2020. p. 173–85.
19. Malamed SF. Recent advances in local anesthesia. In: Handbook of local anesthesia. 7th ed. St. Louis, MO: Elsevier; 2020. p. 367–94.
20. Malamed SF. Supplemental injection techniques. In: Handbook of local anesthesia. 7th ed. St. Louis, MO: Elsevier; 2020. p. 268–88.
21. Fayle SA, Duggal MS. Local analgesia. In: Duggal MS, Curzon MEJ, Fayle SA, Toumba KJ, Robertson AJ, editors. Restorative techniques in pediatric dentistry. 2nd ed. London: Martin Dunitz; 2002. p. 13–27.
22. Mittal M, Sharma S, Kumar A, Chopra R, Srivastava D. Comparison of anesthetic efficacy of articaine and lidocaine during primary maxillary molar extractions in children. Pediatr Dent. 2015;37(7):520–4.
23. Nusstein J, Steinkruger G, Reader A, Beck M, Weaver J. The effects of a 2-stage injection technique on inferior alveolar nerve block injection pain. Anesth Prog. 2006;53:126–30.
24. Joseph RM, Rao AP, Srikant N, Karuna YM, Nayak PA. Comparison of patient comfort during the first stage of conventional versus modified two-stage inferior alveolar nerve blocks in pediatric patients. Anesth Prog. 2019;66(4):221–6. https://doi.org/10.2344/anpr-66-03-03.
25. Fuller NP, Menke RA, Meyers WJ. Perception of pain to three different intraoral penetrations of needles. J Am Dent Assoc. 1979;99:822–4.
26. Ram D, Hemida L, Amir E. Reaction of children to dental injection with 27 or 30 gauge needles. Int J Ped Dent. 2007;17(5):383–7.
27. Ashwin R, Karthik S. A modified two stage technique of administering an inferior alveolar nerve block in children. J Nepal Dent Assoc. 2013;13:139–41.
28. Malamed SF. Anesthetic considerations in dental specialties. In: Handbook of local anesthesia. 7th ed. St. Louis, MO: Elsevier; 2020. p. 289–306.
29. Yu J, Liu S, Zhang X. Can buccal infiltration of articaine replace traditional inferior alveolar nerve block for the treatment of mandibular molars in pediatric patients?: A systematic review and meta-analysis. Med Oral Patol Oral Cir Bucal. 2021;26(6):e754–61. https://doi.org/10.4317/medoral.24726.
30. St George G, Morgan A, Meechan J, Moles DR, Needleman I, Ng YL, Petrie A. Injectable local anaesthetic agents for dental anaesthesia. Cochrane Database Syst Rev. 2018;7(7):CD006487. https://doi.org/10.1002/14651858.CD006487.
31. Arrow P. A comparison of articaine 4% and lignocaine 2% in block and infiltration analgesia in children. Aust Dent J. 2012;57(3):325–33. https://doi.org/10.1111/j.1834-7819.2012.01699.

32. Malamed SF, Tavana S, Falkel M. Faster onset and more comfortable injection with alkalinized 2% lidocaine with epinephrine 1:100,000. Compend Contin Educ Dent. 2013;34:10–20. (Spec No 1).
33. Reed KL, Malamed SF, Fonner AM. Local anesthesia part 2: technical considerations. Anesth Prog. 2012;59(3):127–36; quiz 137. https://doi.org/10.2344/0003-3006-59.3.127.
34. Illusion training and education. Buffering local anesthetic solutions. In: Youtube[IN]. 31 Dec 2016. https://www.youtube.com/watch?v=5BxYfkTDZkM. Accessed 22 Jan 2022.
35. Bokesch PM, Raymond SA, Strichartz GR. Dependence of lidocaine potency on pH and PCO2. Anesth Analg. 1987;66(1):9–17.

Midazolam: A Step-by-Step Clinical Protocol

7

7.1 Overview

A step-by-step protocol provides a channel towards a successful sedation appointment. It also aids the clinician retrospectively evaluate the sedation session for improved future outcomes. Minimal/moderate sedation with midazolam is *unlike* deep sedation or general anesthesia. There will be a lot of "stop and proceed" phases requiring skill, patience, and intelligent clinical maneuvering. A protocol will also help the clinician fine tune this aspect. This chapter will start with a description of the objective signs of sedation, permitting the initiation of treatment. It will further take the reader through a step-by-step clinical protocol of treatment under midazolam. Important issues like parental presence in the operatory, combining midazolam with inhalation sedation, the role of protective stabilization, intraoperative monitoring, local anesthesia, discharge criteria, post-operative instructions, and documentation will also be addressed briefly.

7.2 Background and Objective

We have discussed so far the pre-operative assessment, the case selection based on Frankl behavior rating scale, and the routes of midazolam administration in Chap. 3, Chap. 4, and Chap. 5, respectively. Here, in this chapter, we start the discussion, assuming that appropriate case selection has been done and the child has been administered the prescribed dose of midazolam through one of the available routes, best suited for the child.

The name of the drug, route or site of administration, time of administration, dosage/kilogram, number of ampules of midazolam used (if applicable), and any remarks (e.g., *child expectorated unverifiable quantity of the drug during oral administration*) should be documented in the patient record.

The objective of this chapter will be to guide the reader on the timing of treatment initiation based on the objective signs of sedation and take her/him through the entire step-by-step process of pediatric dental treatment under midazolam sedation.

7.3   The Objective Signs of Sedation

The onset of clinical sedation will vary depending on the route of sedation. The period between the administration of the drug and the attainment of clinical levels of sedation adequate for treatment to start is called the latency period. In young children, the subjective signs may not be reliable or consistent, and the clinician should bank on the objective signs, to signify the right time to shift the child into the operatory. The drug should not be administered inside the operatory (*with the exception of the intravenous route where there is no latency period*), which may increase the child's anxiety. It can be administered in a separate room, playing soothing music with a neat but not loud ambiance. See Chap. 5. Post drug administration, the parent should closely supervise the child. The child should also be discouraged from indulging in active play. This is also a good time to introduce the pulse oximeter to the child. An assistant should observe the child and alert the clinician when necessary.

The objective signs of sedation signifying the onset of clinically active sedation include [1] (Fig. 7.1):

- Distant look and a child who is visibly less active
- Delayed eye movement
- Unable to stand or sit unaided
- Slurred speech
- Light sleep

The time of onset of the sedation should be noted in the patient records.

Fig. 7.1 The objective signs of sedation

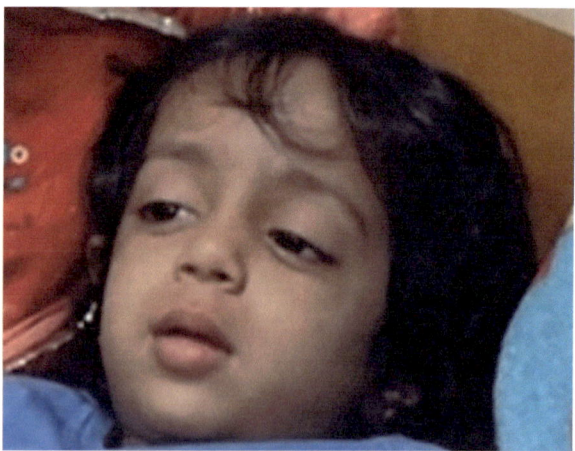

7.4 Parental Presence Inside the Operatory

The parent at this stage carries or assists the child into the operatory and places the child on the already reclined dental chair. The parent can either stay inside the operatory or leave the operatory at this stage, depending on the practice policy. The authors routinely prefer one parent to stay inside the operatory for the following reasons:

- The sedation obtained with midazolam being of a minimal/moderate level means the child, though sedated and relaxed, is still aware of the surrounding environment. The parent suddenly leaving the operatory may unnecessarily induce panic in the child, negating the sedative effects.
- The parent also appreciates firsthand the challenges of child management and the efforts put in by the clinician towards scaling those challenges.

But the groundwork of instructing the parent about not interrupting the communication between the clinician and the child should have already been completed in the informed consent stage.

7.5 "Settling" the Child

Going forward, the next clinical step is to allow the child to "settle" on the dental chair [2]. This is a very important phase the clinician should be aware of. Rushing through to the next steps is often what leads to failure of the sedation appointment. "Settling" emphasizes giving the child sufficient time to calm down on the dental chair before going into the next clinical step. Moderate sedation in general follows a "stop and proceed" approach, which may be done several times through the procedure whenever the clinician senses the child becoming restless or agitated.

7.6 Nitrous Oxide and Oxygen

The use of nitrous oxide-oxygen along with midazolam is a safe and synergistic combination [3]. Midazolam will work to calm the child, decrease anxiety, and facilitate the establishment of two-way communication. This will in turn help introduction and acceptance of the nasal hood [4]. Nitrous oxide-oxygen reinforces the anxiolytic properties of midazolam [5]. It also fills in the deficiencies of midazolam like lack of analgesic properties and a short working time. The analgesic properties and the long working time additionally come with the safety of oxygen.

The combination is especially useful in children displaying negative behavior according to the Frankl's behavior rating scale [6]. The characteristics of these children are explained in detail in Chap. 4. Typically the children with this behavior rating do *not* actively resist treatment but will "whine" or "cry" throughout. They will allow operative treatment, but it will be compromised as they do not follow the instructions. The whine or the cry could either be a coping mechanism for anxiety or an attention-seeking behavior by timid or overprotected children, directed toward the parents. The fear could also stem from a previous unpleasant but, *not a traumatic* dental treatment experience. These children accept the nasal hood. But they *will not keep it stable* nor will they breathe through the nose because of the crying, thus negating the effect of inhalation sedation. The anxiolysis provided by midazolam will calm them and also facilitate the *stability* of the nasal hood. Children with attention-deficit/hyperactivity disorder (ADHD) may also display negative behavior (*according to the Frankl behavior rating scale*) . These children also may *not* actively resist treatment, but their limited attention span does not allow them to keep the nasal hood stable which often hinders ideal treatment.

It is very important for the clinician to understand this concept and differentiate Frankl negative behavior from definitely negative. The children displaying definitely negative behavior *will actively resist* treatment by attempting to leave the dental chair, loud crying, turning the head away, or closing the mouth with their hands. These children *will not accept* the nasal hood or will actively pull it away from their nose. In these children, premedication with midazolam to facilitate the *acceptance* of the nasal hood is *unlikely to succeed*. This is because midazolam in its prescribed dosages is indicated for an anxious child, who is ready to accept the treatment. It calms and helps the child cope up with the stress of the dental treatment. It is not strong enough in prescribed dosages to overcome the strong resistance in a child who is *not* ready to accept the treatment. This child will try to fight the calming effects of midazolam, which may in turn manifest as a paradoxical reaction.

7.7   Protective Stabilization

The use of protective stabilization like a papoose board to restrain the body and extremities depends upon the Frankl rating of the child's behavior. The authors prefer the use of a papoose board for emergency treatment of children displaying definitely negative, subcategory - - 3 behavior. These are the children whose behavior is classified as definitely negative on the Frankl behavior rating scale, displaying disruptive/uncontrolled/combative behavior stemming from true objective fear. They *could* also be children with intellectual and developmental disabilities. Refer to Chap. 4 for an understanding of subcategorization of Frankl definitely negative behavior.

Emergency treatment in the above children can be accomplished with the intramuscular administration (IM) of midazolam at 0.15–0.2 mg/kg body weight. Intranasal midazolam is also an alternative at 0.3–0.4 mg/kg body weight. Midazolam administered through either route creates a short sedation window period, which will help the clinician complete the emergency treatment. Protective stabilization in the form of a papoose board (Fig. 7.2) and molt prop (Fig. 7.3) will help the clinician control the sudden movement of extremities and also aid in mouth opening, to enable local anesthetic administration and subsequent emergency

Fig. 7.2 The papoose board

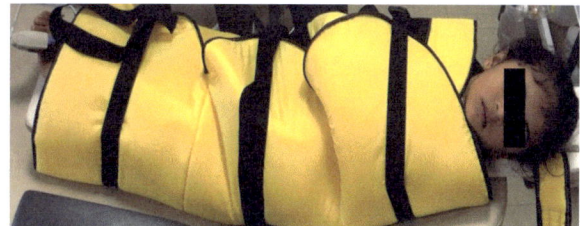

Fig. 7.3 The molt prop

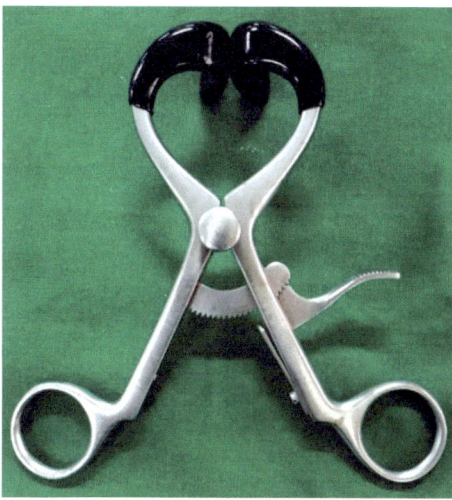

treatment. The anterograde amnesia provided by midazolam will be an added advantage in these scenarios.

For pre-cooperative children below 3 years of age, the authors prefer protective stabilization provided by a parent. The child is placed on the parent's chest with the head lying over the shoulder during treatment. This position provides gentle restraint along with emotional security for the pre-cooperative child (Fig. 7.4).

For children displaying negative or positive behavior (according to Frankl's behavior rating scale), the use of protective stabilization is optional. The question of its role in contributing to the success of minimal/moderate sedation is still open [7]. The papoose board could provide comfort and security to the child, which may further enhance the anxiolytic effect of midazolam. It will also serve to prevent any sudden and unexpected movement of the child. The child if placed on the papoose board should be comfortable with the arms and legs not being tightly squeezed. The child should be able to breathe freely, and the arms, shoulders, and legs should be comfortably extended [2]. It should also allow the placement of monitors as necessary.

Fig. 7.4 Parent on the
dental chair with the
child's head on the parent's
shoulder

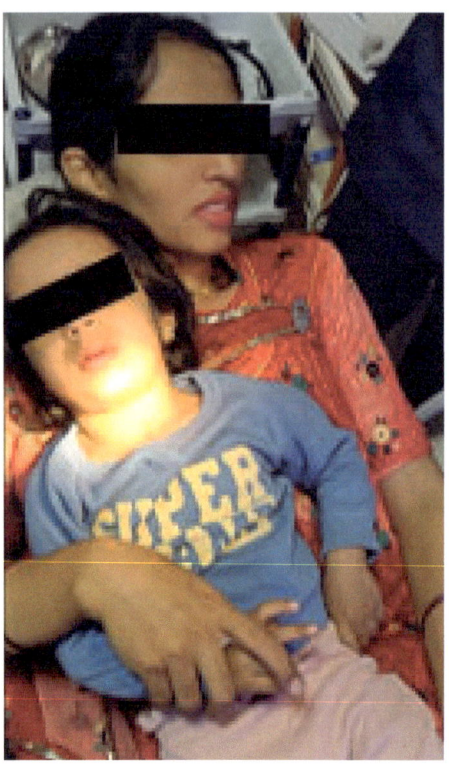

7.8   Personnel and Monitoring

7.8.1   Personnel

Observant personnel and monitoring through appropriate equipment is the standard
of care in sedation. They are especially essential in a child who is sleeping under the
influence of the sedative drug. Stable vital signs and a patent airway are the key
indicators of well-being in a sedated child. In addition to the clinician, moderate
sedation requires a separate PALS (Pediatric Advanced Life Support)-trained individual to monitor the physiologic parameters and to support resuscitation efforts by
the clinician in case of an emergency [8].

7.8.2   Types and Frequency of Monitoring

During the procedure, the level of consciousness, respiratory rate, quality of
breath sounds, heart rate, oxygen saturation, and blood pressure should be

monitored and documented in a time-based record every 10 minutes [8]. The reader is referred to Chap. 9 for a sample of an intraoperative time-based sedation record. According to the American Dental Association, vital signs should be recorded at five stages [9]:

1. Pre-operative for a baseline comparison
2. Intraoperative after drug administration
3. Inter-operative every 10 minutes
4. Immediate post-operative
5. Prior to discharge

7.8.3 Level of Consciousness

Continuous clinical monitoring is imperative with any level of sedation. There are numerous validated sedation rating scales to monitor the level of consciousness with their pluses and shortcomings [10–13]. The authors prefer the "University of Michigan Sedation Scale" for its simplicity and practicality in the clinical setting [10, 14] (Fig. 7.5).

Also recorded is the behavior of the child on a time-based chart according to the following scale [15]:

Excellent: quiet and cooperative
Good: mild objections and/or whimpering but treatment not interrupted
Fair: crying with minimal disruption to treatment
Poor: struggling that interfered with operative procedures
Prohibitive: active resistance and crying; treatment cannot be rendered

Value	Patient state
0	Awake and alert
1	Minimally sedated; tired/sleepy, appropriate response to verbal conversation, and/or sound
2	Moderately sedated: somnolent/sleeping, easily aroused with light tactile stimulation or a simple verbal command
3	Deeply sedated: deep sleep, aroused only with significant physical stimulation
4	Unarousable

Fig. 7.5 University of Michigan sedation scale

7.8.4   Monitoring Equipment

Monitoring equipment compares the baseline vital signs to the values obtained when the child is under sedation. Monitoring equipment for moderate sedation commonly includes a precordial stethoscope, pulse oximeter, and a blood pressure recording apparatus. Recording the expired carbon dioxide values through capnography is recommended where feasible.

7.8.4.1 Precordial Stethoscope

Stethoscopes monitor the heart and respiratory sounds. The respiratory sounds are heard best at the precordial notch. The precordial notch is immediately above the manubrium of the chest. An imaginary triangle is constructed connecting the nipples forming the base with the apex at the precordial notch [2] (Fig. 7.6).

The heart sounds are heard best as the bell is moved from the precordial notch along the imaginary line towards the left nipple. See Chap. 3 for a detailed explanation of the auscultation of the heart and lungs.

The stethoscope monitors two key elements, the rate of breathing (respiratory rate) and the quality of breath sounds.

Breaths are counted for 15 seconds and multiplied by 4 to calculate the rate of breathing in a minute. The rate of breathing varies with age (Fig. 7.7).

The purpose of measuring the rate of breathing is to detect tachypnea (rapid rate of breathing) or bradypnea (very slow rate of breathing).

The quality of good breath sounds indicates a patent airway with normal unobstructed airflow heard as "whooshing" sound on the stethoscope. Normal respiratory sounds serve as a reassurance to the clinician that the airway is open and clear of debris. Partial airway obstruction is signified through various sounds like

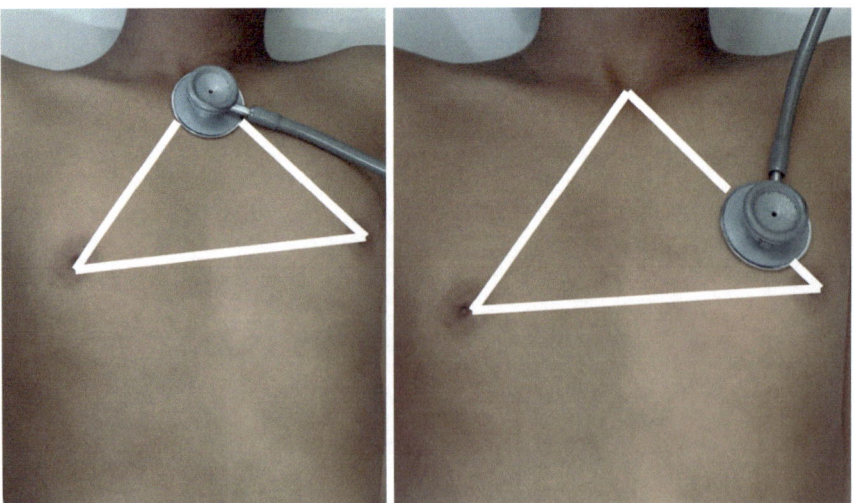

Fig. 7.6   Best areas to hear the respiratory and heart sounds

Fig. 7.7 Respiratory rate
at various ages

AGE (In Years)	RATE (Breaths/Minute)
Below 1	30-40
2-5	25-30
6-12	20-25
Above 12	15-20

Sound	Cause	Management
Snoring	Obstruction by the tongue	Head tilt chin lift
Gurgling	Foreign matter in the airway like blood, vomitus, water	Suction the airway
Wheezing	Bronchospasm	Bronchodilator
Crowing	Partial laryngospasm	Suction airway and administer positive pressure oxygen

Fig. 7.8 Causes of partial airway obstruction

snoring, gurgling, wheezing, or crowing. See Fig. 7.8 for the significance and early management of partial air obstruction [9].

Silence in the earpiece signifies complete respiratory obstruction (in the presence of exaggerated chest movements) or respiratory arrest (no chest movements). The use of the stethoscope allows early recognition of partial or complete airway obstructions, thus facilitating early corrective measures.

7.8.4.2 Bluetooth Stethoscope
A Bluetooth stethoscope with a transmitter on the bell and a receiver fitting the ears of the monitoring personnel transmits the sound wirelessly over several feet. This allows the monitoring personnel more freedom of movement. The signal can also be turned off if required with the push of a button.

7.8.4.3 The Pulse Oximeter
Clinically, the pale color of the mucosa, skin, or blood can potentially indicate desaturation. But these are late indicators. The pulse oximeter on the other hand continuously monitors the pulse rate and blood oxygen saturation percentage

Fig. 7.9 Wrap-around
pulse oximeter sensor

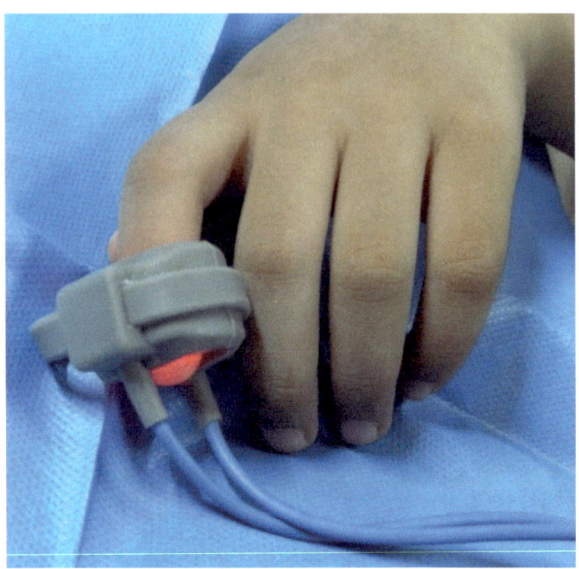

and provides an early warning during the event of a desaturation. The pulse oximeter probe can be attached on the finger or the big toe of the child. At sea level, the acceptable percentage of oxygen saturation ranges from 95 to 99%. The acceptable range can decrease at higher sea levels. Adhesive or wrap-around sensors may be used if the child does not stably retain the clip-on sensors (Fig. 7.9).

7.8.4.4 The Sphygmomanometer

The width of the blood pressure cuff selected should be two-thirds the length of the upper arm, between the shoulder and the elbow joints. It should fit snug and not too tight on the child's upper left arm. The child should have been already exposed to the experience of inflation during the pre-operative assessment. The experience should not be initiated first time when the child is under sedation, as it may alarm the child. If the inflation of the blood pressure cuff causes agitation in the child making it unfeasible, this should be documented in the patient's chart.

7.8.4.5 Capnography

Capnography reinforces the information provided by the stethoscope in a child sleeping under the influence of a sedative drug. It is not useful in a moving or crying child. The capnograph monitor displays waveforms, representing the expired carbon dioxide. Diminished height of the waveforms in a sleeping child may indicate a partially blocked airway.

7.9   Administration of Local Anesthesia

Midazolam elevates the pain threshold and modifies the perception and reaction of the child towards the pain. It does not provide actual pain control due to the lack of analgesic properties. That has to be controlled with the administration of local anesthesia [16]. Local anesthesia should be administered very gently, ideally with zero discomfort. Pain during the injection process will alert the child decreasing the anti-anxiety and sedative effect of midazolam. It may even lead to a paradoxical reaction [17]. On the other hand, local anesthesia administered *without* the child experiencing pain, deepens the calmness and the relaxation produced by midazolam. Hence, this is a critical phase in the midazolam sedation episode. The administration of local anesthesia in children with minimal discomfort involves a process in addition to specific techniques and clinical considerations. This aspect is described in detail in Chap. 6. A common error during the administration of local anesthesia in a sedated child is the tendency of the clinician to block the nostrils during the administration of the supraperiosteal injection to the maxillary anterior teeth. This could lead to desaturation and the clinician should be alert to this (Fig. 7.10).

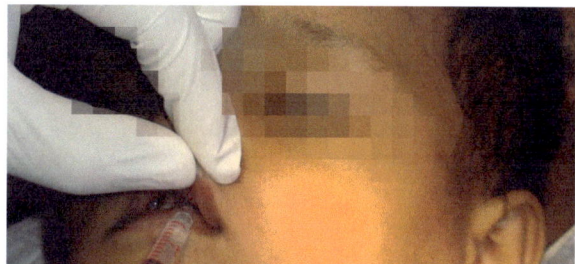

Fig. 7.10 Tendency for the nostrils to be blocked during injection near the maxillary anterior teeth

7.10   Rubber Dam Application for Restorative Procedures

Rubber dam is the standard of care in restorative dentistry. In moderate sedation, the consciousness is depressed with the potential possibility of a compromised swallowing reflex. Hence, the application of rubber dam becomes even more imperative during procedures under sedation. In addition to providing isolation and preventing soft tissue injuries, it also protects the airway against the accidental ingestion or aspiration of foreign bodies including water from the high-speed airotor handpiece, restorative materials, or crowns. In fact, the use of rubber dam has shown to promote more positive behavior in children under moderate sedation compared to other isolation methods like IsoVac [18]. Local anesthesia facilitates the placement of the rubber dam clamps. Dental floss should be secured to the clamp on either side of the bow as a safety measure against unexpected fracture or dislodgement of the clamp. Quadrant isolation of each tooth separately should be preferred to the slit dam technique. Also in the lower arch, quadrant isolation should be preferred over arch isolation where there is a possibility of pushing the tongue further posteriorly towards the pharynx.

Two important clinical points that should be emphasized at this stage, on a separate note independent to the discussion on rubber dam, are the following:

- The clinician should be conscious of the child's head tilt-chin lift at all times during the restorative procedure. This is especially important while working on the mandibular arch where there will be a tendency to push the mandible down towards the chest, potentially compromising the airway.
- In the case of extraction, in a pre-cooperative child, absorbable hemostatic sponges are very useful compared to the sterile gauze, to control hemorrhage. This is because of the possibility of the young sedated child swallowing the gauze.

7.11   Discharge Criteria

At the end of the procedure, the child should not be rushed into a sitting position which may lead to orthostatic hypotension. The child also should not be allowed to walk without parent support as she/he is led to the recovery area. Monitoring should continue till discharge. The recovery area should be equipped with facility to deliver 100% oxygen, suction apparatus, and a bag valve mask device to deliver positive pressure ventilation. The discharge criteria include:

- The child should be responding to her/his name (if age appropriate)
- The child should sit up unaided (if age appropriate) without dizziness
- There should be no signs of disorientation
- The vital signs should be close to the baseline values

– The pre-sedation level of responsiveness should have been observed. For a very young child or a child with disability incapable of the usual expected response, a level as close as possible to the pre-sedation level should be confirmed.
– The child's ability to stay awake for 20 minutes (University of Michigan Sedation Scale, value 0) in a quiet environment is also a simple evaluation tool to determine discharge [19].

7.12   Post-Operative Instructions to Parents

Post-operative parent instructions include:

– Medication instructions
– Transport of the child from the treatment facility to home
– Feeding instructions
– Monitoring the child over the next 24 hours

Antibiotics and analgesics as necessary can be prescribed. The parents should be warned about the soft tissue numbness post local anesthesia and possibility of lip biting.

Two adults should accompany the child home. One should be in charge of driving the vehicle, and the other caregiver/parent should be monitoring the child. Should the child wish to sleep on the way home, this caregiver or parent should keep the airway open with the chin off the chest and a head tilt.

Once home, the child should be started initially on clear fluids. If the child accepts it well, soft food can be started in small portions. Large portions and fatty foods should be avoided. The child should be well hydrated for the next 24 hours.

The parents should be made aware that the child could sleep more, in the next 24-hours period. During sleep, the child should be on her/his side left lateral position and not in the supine position. Pillows can be placed on the back and the abdomen to stabilize the child in this position. The parents should be warned against placing the pillow near the child's face. Parents should periodically monitor the sleeping child in general and specifically for any episodes of vomiting. When awake, the child should not be playing alone and should always be under close adult supervision. The child may be unsteady or dizzy, and activities like bicycle riding or climbing stairs will be a strict no-no. The child could also be irritable for 24 hours.

The instructions should be given orally and reinforced with written documentation. See Chap. 9 for an annexure on discharge criteria and post-operative instructions. It is always a good practice for the clinician to call the parents within 24 hours and inquire about the child.

Clinically Relevant Points

1. Post drug administration, in young children, the subjective signs may not be reliable or consistent, and the clinician should bank on the objective signs to signify the right time to shift the child into the operatory.
2. The authors routinely prefer one parent to stay inside the operatory during the treatment of the child under sedation.
3. "Settling" the child implies giving the child sufficient time to calm down before commencing the treatment.
4. The use of nitrous oxide-oxygen along with midazolam is a safe and synergistic combination.
5. The use of protective stabilization during minimal/moderate sedation depends on the Frankl behavior rating of the child.
6. The "University of Michigan Sedation Scale" is a simple and practical scale to monitor the level of consciousness.
7. Monitoring equipment for moderate sedation commonly includes a precordial stethoscope, pulse oximeter, and a blood pressure recording apparatus.
8. Local anesthesia should be administered very gently, ideally with zero discomfort to the child during midazolam sedation. Pain during the injection process will alert the child decreasing the antianxiety and sedative effect of midazolam. It may even lead to a paradoxical reaction.
9. The child's ability to stay awake for 20 minutes in a quiet environment is also a simple evaluation tool to determine discharge.
10. Should the child wish to sleep on the way home, this caregiver or parent should keep the airway open with the chin off the chest and a head tilt.

References

1. Smith BM, Cutilli BJ, Saunders W. Oral midazolam: pediatric conscious sedation. Compend Contin Educ Dent. 1998;19(6):586–8, 590, 592l
2. Wilson S. Protocol. In: Wilson S, editor. Oral sedation for dental procedures in children. Berlin: Springer; 2015. p. 113–39.
3. Litman RS, Berkowitz RJ, Ward DS. Levels of consciousness and ventilatory parameters in young children during sedation with oral midazolam and nitrous oxide. Arch Pediatr Adolesc Med. 1996;150(7):671–5. https://doi.org/10.1001/archpedi.1996.02170320017002.
4. Sivaramakrishnan G, Sridharan K. Nitrous oxide and midazolam sedation: a systematic review and meta-analysis. Anesth Prog. 2017;64(2):59–65. https://doi.org/10.2344/anpr-63-03-06.
5. Berge TI. Acceptance and side effects of nitrous oxide oxygen sedation for oral surgical procedures. Acta Odontol Scand. 1999;57(4):201–6. https://doi.org/10.1080/000163599428788.
6. Al-Zahrani AM, Wyne AH, Sheta SA. Comparison of oral midazolam with a combination of oral midazolam and nitrous oxide-oxygen inhalation in the effectiveness of dental

sedation for young children. J Indian Soc Pedod Prev Dent. 2009;27(1):9–16. https://doi.org/10.4103/0970-4388.50810.

7. Shapira J, Kupietzky A, Kadari A, Fuks AB, Holan G. Comparison of oral midazolam with and without hydroxyzine in the sedation of pediatric dental patients. Pediatr Dent. 2004;26(6):492–6.

8. Coté CJ, Wilson S. Guidelines for monitoring and management of pediatric patients before, during, and after sedation for diagnostic and therapeutic procedures. Pediatr Dent. 2019;41(4):259–60.

9. Malamed SF. Monitoring during sedation. In: 6th ed., editor. Sedation: a guide to patient management. St. Louis, MO: Elsevier; 2018. p. 66–85.

10. Malviya S, Voepel-Lewis T, Tait AR, Merkel S, Tremper K, Naughton N. Depth of sedation in children undergoing computed tomography: validity and reliability of the University of Michigan Sedation Scale (UMSS). Br J Anaesth. 2002;88(2):241–5. https://doi.org/10.1093/bja/88.2.241.

11. Ramsay MA, Savege TM, Simpson BR, Goodwin R. Controlled sedation with alphaxalone-alphadolone. Br Med J. 1974;2(5920):656–9. https://doi.org/10.1136/bmj.2.5920.656.

12. Agrawal D, Feldman HA, Krauss B, Waltzman ML. Bispectral index monitoring quantifies depth of sedation during emergency department procedural sedation and analgesia in children. Ann Emerg Med. 2004;43(2):247–55. https://doi.org/10.1016/s0196-0644(03)00721-2.

13. Ghajari MF, Ansari G, Hasanbeygi L, Shayeghi S. Conscious sedation efficacy of 0.3 and 0.5 mg/kg oral midazolam for three to six year-old uncooperative children undergoing dental treatment: a clinical trial. J Dent (Tehran). 2016;13(2):101–7.

14. Kim EJ, Jo YY, Kil HK. Optimal sedative dose of propofol to start MRI in children with cerebral palsy. Korean J Anesthesiol. 2011;61(3):216–9. https://doi.org/10.4097/kjae.2011.61.3.216.

15. Sedation Record. https://www.aapd.org/globalassets/media/policies_guidelines/r_sedationrecord.pdf. Accessed 23 April 2022.

16. Alzahrani AM, Wyne AH. Use of oral midazolam sedation in pediatric dentistry: a review. Pak Oral Dent J. 2012;32(3):444–55.

17. Malamed SF. Pharmacology. In: Sedation: a guide to patient management. 6th ed. St. Louis, MO: Elsevier; 2018. p. 319–58.

18. Current JL, Unkel JH, Berry EJ, Reinhartz J, Reinhartz D. Comparing behavior outcomes with rubber dam or IsoVac isolation in patients undergoing moderate sedation. J Dent Child (Chic). 2022;89(2):83–7.

19. Malviya S, Voepel-Lewis T, Ludomirsky A, Marshall J, Tait AR. Can we improve the assessment of discharge readiness?: a comparative study of observational and objective measures of depth of sedation in children. Anesthesiology. 2004;100(2):218–24. https://doi.org/10.1097/00000542-200402000-00007.

SAFE: Sedation Attitudes to Forestall Emergencies

8

8.1 Overview

Sedation Attitudes to Forestall Emergencies acronymed **SAFE** conveys that clinicians should develop an attitude, respecting the ground rules governing the safe practice of sedation to prevent emergencies. The first part of the chapter elaborates on these ground rules. The latter part of the chapter specifically explains the management of sedation-related emergencies. It also gives a list of the emergency equipment and drugs recommended by the authors, suitable for a dental office practicing minimal/moderate sedation in children.

8.2 Background and Objective

"When you prepare for an emergency, the emergency ceases to exist" [1]. An important part of this preparation involves an awareness that emergencies occur and occur when least expected. Developing an attitude where the ground rules for sedation are respected and followed, will aid the clinician a long way in forestalling these emergencies. But, despite precautions, sedation-related emergencies still happen, and the clinician has to respond appropriately during this high-stake occurrence. A simple, well-familiarized emergency kit with only the necessary drugs and equipment and a simple protocol will help the clinician think clearly during an emergency and enable the rescue of the child. The latter part of the chapter will focus on emergency management related to minimal/moderate sedation in a pediatric dental setting.

8.3   Ground Rules Governing the Safe Practice of Sedation in Pediatric Dentistry

These rules are broadly based on recommendations from the *"Guidelines for Monitoring and Management of Pediatric Patients Before, During, and After Sedation for Diagnostic and Therapeutic Procedures"* [2]. These include:

1. A meticulous pre-operative assessment
2. A strict "nil per oral" (*NPO*) compliance
3. "Single drug-single dose" rule for minimal/moderate sedation
4. Understanding the difference between minimal, moderate, and deep sedation and general anesthesia
5. Following the recommended monitoring, personnel, and infrastructure protocols for the planned level of sedation
6. Following the recovery and discharge protocols

8.3.1   A Meticulous Pre-operative Assessment

The ultimate objective of a pre-operative assessment is to help the clinician classify the child under the *American Society of Anesthesiologists (ASA)* classification indicating the systemic status of a child. Depending on the ASA classification, the clinician makes the decision to post the child for treatment under sedation as an outpatient in the dental office or in the hospital setup. Only ASA I and ASA II children can be taken up for sedation safely in the dental office [3].

To arrive at an ASA category for the child, seven aspects have to be recorded and analyzed:

1. A structured medical history
2. Evaluation of vital signs
3. Body mass index (BMI) for age percentiles
4. Tonsil size and extraoral anatomic abnormalities
5. Mallampati classification for the child
6. History of upper respiratory tract infection (URTI)
7. Auscultation of the lungs and heart

The reader is referred to Chap. 3 for a detailed description on pre-operative assessment.

8.3.2   Strict "Nil per Oral" (*NPO*) Compliance

Pulmonary aspiration of food can be potentially a life-threatening emergency during a sedation episode should the child become nauseous and vomit. Though highly unlikely in minimal/moderate sedation as the protective reflexes are intact by definition, the parents should still be explained about this potential complication during the pre-sedation appointment. NPO has additional significance during oral sedation where failure to comply with the NPO protocol will cause inadequate absorption of the drug.

8.3.2.1 The NPO Protocol

The conventional NPO protocol follows a simple 2-4-6-8 rule. Clear fluids should be avoided within 2 hours of the administration of the sedative drug. Breast milk should be avoided within 4 hours, light meals including non-human milk within 6 hours, and fatty meals within 8 hours.

8.3.2.2 Practical NPO for Minimal/Moderate Sedation

NPO before minimal/moderate sedation in a young child has to be balanced out with its ill effects, namely, hypoglycemia, electrolyte imbalance, and dehydration. It should be remembered that unlike deep sedation or general anesthesia, the child will not receive additional intravenous fluids during minimal/moderate sedation. This could lead the child to become irritated resulting in an undesirable paradoxical reaction. The child is therefore permitted unlimited amounts of clear fluids 2 hours before sedative administration. This recommendation is based on the fact that clear fluids are rapidly emptied from the stomach. In fact, the updated guidelines by the European Society for Paediatric Anaesthesiology (ESPA) endorsed by the Society for Paediatric Anesthesia of Australia and New Zealand encourage drinking clear fluids till 1 hour prior to surgery, in elective surgery, unless specific contraindications exist [4]. Carbohydrate-rich clear fluids (e.g., *pulp-free clear apple juice, "Appy," Parle Agro Pvt. Ltd., Maharashtra, India*) at volumes ranging from 3 mL/kg to 5 mL/kg body weight have been recommended [5, 6].

8.3.2.3 Clear Fluids

It should clearly be mentioned to parents on what comprises clear fluids. Clear fluids include water, fruit juice without pulp or particulate matter, carbonated drinks, and tea or coffee without milk [7]. Milk should be avoided because it coagulates in the acidic environment of the stomach and delays gastric emptying. To simplify the concept of clear fluids further to the parents, it can also be explained that, if poured in a transparent glass and held up to a bright light source, the light source should be seen through the clear fluids [8].

8.3.3 "Single Drug-Single Dose"

"Single drug-single dose" of a sedative implies that a single drug should be used to obtain minimal/moderate sedation with a single dose. The use of multiple drugs or multiple doses can potentially lead to life-threatening emergencies [9].

8.3.3.1 A "Single" Drug

A cocktail or combination of drugs in an ideal scenario would be a mixture of two or more sedative drugs where a pharmacological shortcoming in the sedative characteristic of one drug would be made up by the other drug. For example, the lack of analgesic properties of midazolam can be made up by adding meperidine. Though there are advantages to this concept, the doses have to be carefully adjusted to prevent unintended deeper levels of sedation. As has been emphasized in this book, midazolam at prescribed doses in conjunction with non-pharmacological behavior management methods and effective local anesthetic techniques results in predictable minimal/moderate sedation more often than not. An exception to the "single drug" rule is the use of midazolam along with nitrous oxide-oxygen. Midazolam combines well and safely with nitrous oxide-oxygen, which provides additional advantages of supplemental oxygen, analgesia, and a prolonged working time [10, 11].

Also, when a single drug is used to obtain minimal/moderate sedation, it is better to use a drug whose *primary* pharmacological action is sedation, e.g., midazolam. The independent use of drugs like hydroxyzine or meperidine should be avoided. This is because these drugs are not primarily intended for sedation. Sedation is their secondary pharmacological effect, which gets activated at higher doses potentially leading to complications.

8.3.3.2 A "Single" Dose

The "single dose" rule is applicable to non-titratable routes of sedation. With midazolam, this therefore applies to all the routes except the intravenous route. The disadvantage of non-titratable routes is that a bolus dose is administered based on the child's weight. There will be a latency period before the sedative action of the drug is seen. Hence, the dose cannot be titrated to the ideal clinical effect.

> Latency period is the time occurring between the administrations and the onset of clinical action of the drug.

Titration by Appointment

In non-titratable routes of drug administration, at a given recommended drug dose calculated based on weight, most of the children will display the desired sedative effect. But a small percentage of children remain under-sedated. In this scenario, the second dose should not be administered. The planned clinical procedure should be aborted, and the clinician could increase the drug dose in the subsequent appointment. This concept is called "titration by appointment" [12]. "Titration by appointment" precludes administration of the second dose of the drug in the same appointment and adds to the safety profile of the sedation procedure.

Expectoration of the Drug by the Child
In the event that the child expectorates the drug partially (*as in oral administration*), the clinician should not try and guess the amount of drug that may have been absorbed and administer the second dose. There are two courses of action that can be followed in this scenario. The first is to wait for the latency period to tide over. It may turn out that the partial dose administered to the child provides adequate sedation allowing the clinician to complete the planned procedure. In case the child remains under-sedated, the clinician may opt for another route in the next appointment, like the intranasal route, to reliably administer the planned dosage of the drug.

8.3.4   Understanding Deep Sedation/General Anesthesia and Moderate Sedation

8.3.4.1 Deep Sedation
The novice clinician sometimes administers sedative drugs that put the child in a deep state of sedation. The child in this state floats between the semiconscious and the unconscious state. The clinician may feel a false sense of elation for having calmed the child enough to render operative treatment. This is impending disaster due to the inexperience of the clinician. It is important to realize that the child here, for all practical purposes, is in general anesthesia. Deep sedation and general anesthesia are a continuum, and the terminology or definitions are only academic. In deep sedation, the child is in Guedel stage 1 of anesthesia or in the ultra-light plane of general anesthesia [13]. The monitoring, the infrastructure, and the personnel required in this case are on par with general anesthesia requirements [2]. It is once again emphasized that the child in deep sedation is practically unconscious unless a deeply painful stimulus occurs. It is only a step away from general anesthesia where the child will be continually unconscious and unresponsive to any degree of painful stimuli.

8.3.4.2 The Induction of General Anesthesia with Intravenous Drugs
The difference or rather a lack of clinical difference between deep sedation and general anesthesia should be very clear to the clinician practicing sedation in Pediatric Dentistry. One common misconception among inexperienced clinicians is that general anesthesia involves the use of gases for induction, whereas the intravenous administration of drugs is sedation. The clinician should be aware of the technique acronymed "TIVA" (*total intravenous anesthesia*) where general anesthesia is completely induced and maintained intravenously.

8.3.4.3 Airway Management in General Anesthesia
Another misconception is that general anesthesia compulsorily requires endotracheal intubation. If an open airway (***NO airway adjunct*** *like an endotracheal tube or a LMA protecting the glottis)* is present, then it is assumed to be sedation. This is

again not the case. General anesthesia by definition is "A drug induced loss of consciousness during which patients are not arousable, even by painful stimulation. The ability to independently maintain ventilatory function is often impaired. *Patients often require assistance in maintaining a patent airway* and positive pressure ventilation may be required because of depressed spontaneous ventilation or drug induced depression of neuromuscular function. Cardiovascular function may be impaired" [2]. Let us focus our attention on the underlined part of the above definition, which stresses the need for "*assistance in maintaining a patent airway.*" It should be noted that "assistance to maintaining a patent airway" could imply the use of just the basic nasopharyngeal tube. It does not imply the mandatory use of advanced airway management devices like the laryngeal mask airway or endotracheal intubation. Intubation is absolutely necessary only when the child is in an aspiration risk as in a long dental operatory procedure or the child where NPO has been compromised. Intubation secures the airway against aspiration in the above scenarios as further explained in the next paragraph. General anesthesia is the loss of consciousness caused by the administration of drugs regardless of the method of airway management.

8.3.4.4 Airway Management for Dental Restorative Procedures Under Deep Sedation/General Anesthesia

When a child is semiconscious or unconscious as in deep sedation or general anesthesia, the cough reflex and the swallowing reflexes are partially or completely absent. This potentially predisposes the child to aspiration and/or laryngospasm due to irritation of the airway by the foreign bodies (debris, water, saliva, blood, etc.) generated during the dental operative procedures. This is why, ideally, the airway needs to be secured with endotracheal intubation for long dental operatory procedures under general anesthesia. Deep sedation (light planes of general anesthesia) with an open airway should be reserved only for extremely short dental procedures with judicious use of water [14] and careful placement of the rubber dam. The split rubber dam method is best avoided in these scenarios.

8.3.4.5 Understanding the Implications of the Loss of Muscle Tone in Deep Sedation/General Anesthesia

An unconscious or semiconscious child may lose the skeletal muscle tone in the tongue and the upper airway, leading to physical blockage and collapse of the airway. Let us understand the implications of this by drawing a comparison with "obstructive sleep apnea" (OSA).

The loss of skeletal muscle tone with the tongue falling posteriorly in fact may even happen during deep sleep. This is especially true in children predisposed to obstructive sleep apnea (OSA). In OSA, the anatomic abnormalities leading to a narrow airway along with the loss of muscle tone that occurs in the rapid eye movement (REM) sleep lead to partial or complete obstruction of the upper airway. This obstruction results in brief arousal of the child from sleep. Arousal from sleep is accompanied by the regaining of the muscle tone and return of spontaneous ventilation. These cycles of obstruction followed by arousal and the regaining of the muscular tone form the pathophysiological basis of obstructive sleep apnea. A similar loss of muscle tone occurs in deep sedation/general anesthesia as well. But the difference here is that the child may not wake up and regain the muscle tone. The lack of arousal compounded by the loss of protective reflexes and the decrease in the central respiratory drive leading to shallow breathing (*respiratory depression*) with their dangerous implications are the reasons why the untrained clinician should not venture into unintended deep sedation or general anesthesia.

8.3.4.6 Differentiating Deep Sedation/General Anesthesia from Moderate Sedation

Let us examine the definition of moderate sedation first. "Moderate sedation (old terminology, "conscious sedation") is a drug-induced depression of consciousness during which patients respond purposefully to verbal commands or after light tactile stimulation. No interventions are required to maintain a patent airway, and spontaneous ventilation is adequate. Cardiovascular function is usually maintained. The caveat that loss of consciousness should be unlikely is a particularly important aspect of the definition of moderate sedation; drugs and techniques used should carry a margin of safety wide enough to render unintended loss of consciousness unlikely" [2].

The definition implies that moderate sedation is essentially a "conscious" technique. The child remains conscious throughout the sedation episode. A brief closure of eyes or sleep is easily interrupted with a light tactile stimulation like a tap on the shoulder. The child may also show a "purposeful" reaction to a painful stimulus like a local anesthetic injection by crying or trying to push the syringe away.

The definition of moderate sedation also emphasizes that "no interventions are required to maintain a patent airway and spontaneous ventilation is adequate." This lack of intervention to open the airway includes even the most basic chin lift/jaw thrust maneuver [15]. The chin lift/jaw thrust maneuver during sedation is commonly used when the clinician observes a small drop in oxygen saturation and diagnoses it to be from the obstruction caused by the falling back of the tongue. A child under moderate sedation should not require even this basic intervention. A light tap on the shoulder by calling out her/his name should be sufficient to arouse her/him and regain the muscle tone of the tongue stimulating spontaneous ventilation.

The last part of the definition says "drugs and techniques used should carry a margin of safety wide enough to render unintended loss of consciousness unlikely."

Let us understand the concept of moderate sedation drugs through Fig. 8.1.

In the above figure representing moderate sedation, "A weak boy" is seen trying to lift "A heavy weight" and is unable to do it. So now, if the heavy weight is considered to be the child's resistance and the weak boy to be the moderate sedation drug, then what the picture conveys is that "*The moderate sedation drug is too weak to overcome the child's strong resistance*." So, essentially, that means moderate sedation drugs, at average recommended dosages, will not be able to overcome strong resistance in a child displaying combative/uncontrolled/hysterical/disruptive behavior (*See* Chap. 4). Moderate sedation drugs like midazolam (*at recommended dosages*) will be most effective in an anxious/tense cooperative child but, who is

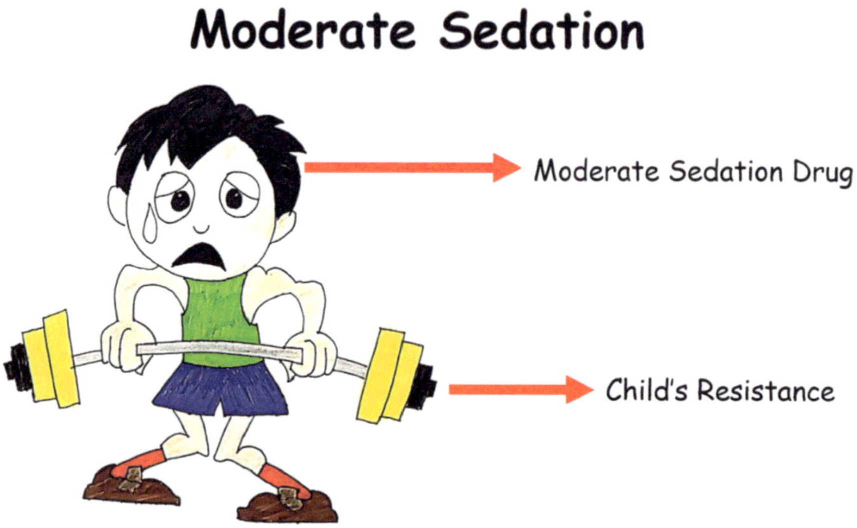

Moderate Sedation

Moderate Sedation Drug

Child's Resistance

Fig. 8.1 Depiction of moderate sedation drugs

ready to accept the treatment. and will go hand in hand with sound basic behavior guidance methods [16]. Moderate sedation drugs will help the child cope up with the stress of the dental treatment but will not be able to override extreme negative behavior.

So, as a good practice, the clinician should categorize the child's behavior and make the early decision to use moderate sedation if the child displays tense cooperative (anxious) or positive or negative behavior according to Frankl behavior rating scale. The clinician should not delay the sedation decision too long to the point where the child develops definitely negative behavior of a combative/uncontrolled/ hysterical/disruptive nature. At this stage, moderate sedation will be ineffective. The child at this stage will require deep sedation or general anesthesia. Here, an anesthesiologist will come into the picture and use heavy-duty drugs like ketamine, propofol, fentanyl, and sevoflurane among others in various combinations, to overcome the child's resistance. As depicted in Fig. 8.2, the deep sedation drugs are strong enough to override any intensity of child resistance.

8.3.5 Following the Recommended Monitoring, Personnel, and Infrastructure Protocols for the Planned Level of Sedation

The purpose of monitoring is to provide the clinician with a warning or an alert, when there is a change in the recommended physiological parameters in a sedated child. The monitoring can be clinical as in an alert assistant who may observe changes in the breathing pattern of the child or through tools like a stethoscope or a

Deep Sedation

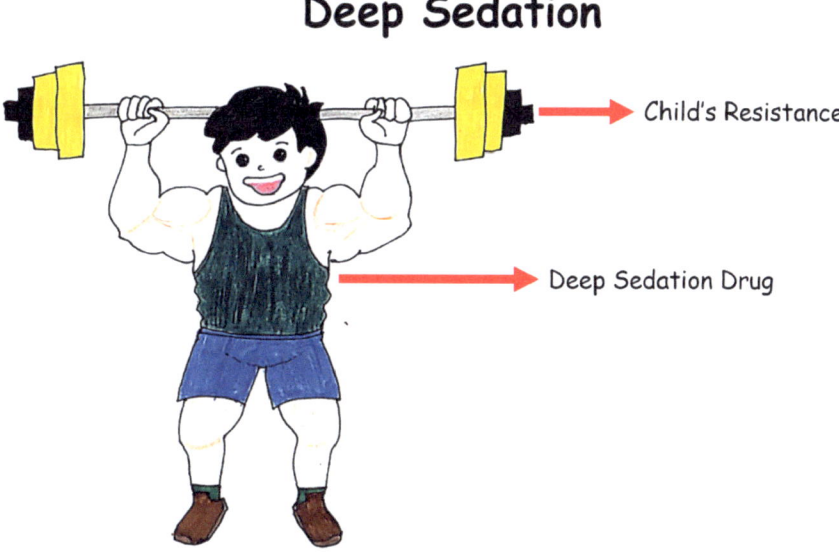

Child's Resistance

Deep Sedation Drug

Fig. 8.2 Depiction of deep sedation/general anesthesia drugs

pulse oximeter. The AAPD recommendations clearly outline the monitoring and infrastructure requirements for the different levels of sedation [2]. The reader is referred to Chap. 7 for a more elaborate description of monitoring during moderate sedation.

8.3.6   Following the Recovery and Discharge Protocols

The clinician can ill afford to be negligent post the operative care of the child under sedation. There could be a tendency to let the guard down after the successful completion of a challenging dental procedure under sedation. A recovery area, following the recommended discharge criteria and detailed post-operative notes including feeding instructions and parental supervision till the child is back to full fitness, ensures the smooth completion of the sedation episode. The reader is referred to Chap. 7 for an elaborate discussion of the same.

8.4   Management of Sedation-Related Emergencies

8.4.1   The Two Potential Complications of Moderate Sedation

When the child (ASA I or II) progresses from a stage of moderate sedation towards deep sedation, two common complications can occur:

- The obstruction of the airway, secondary to loss of the muscle tone
- Hypoventilation (respiratory depression) secondary to drug overdose, due to loss of the central respiratory drive

These airway complications are the primary initiating events, which can lead to subsequent secondary life-threatening cardiac complications like bradycardia and subsequent cardiac arrest if not recognized and managed early.

8.4.2   Basic Management of Desaturation in a Deeply Sedated Child

Deep sedation may be suspected early if the child is unresponsive to verbal and tactile stimulation. Decreased oxygenation in a deeply sedated child may be detected by clinical observation of the child, diminished breath sounds heard in the stethoscope, inadequate end tidal carbon dioxide, or inadequate oxygen saturation displayed by the pulse oximeter.

The decreased oxygenation could commonly be due to:

- Improper positioning of the child's head on the dental chair
- Pooling of saliva in the throat
- Working on the mandibular arch, thereby applying pressure and pushing it back
- Tongue falling back and physically obstructing the airway

Simple measures of airway management in these cases can be initiated by placing the child supine with legs elevated slightly with a pillow. A shoulder roll is placed to raise the torso, the airway is suctioned, and a head tilt-chin lift or a jaw thrust is done. Nitrous oxide if being used is reduced, and the mixture dial is turned to 100% oxygen. Alternatively, supplemental 100% oxygen can be administered via a face mask. The child may become responsive with these measures within 1–3 min. The saturation may also improve with these measures though there will be a short time lag before the oxygen saturation increase is seen in the pulse oximeter.

8.4.3   Diagnosing the Complication and Management in a Continued Desaturation Scenario

In spite of these measures, if the saturation continues to fall, with the child becoming difficult to arouse, the clinician should be alerted to a possible potential life-threatening respiratory emergency. Bibs, papoose board, the garments, or anything covering the child's chest should be cleared, to enable clinical observation of the breathing pattern.

A rocking horse movement or paradoxical breathing pattern, characterized by an alternate rise and fall of the chest and abdomen, respectively, with no airway movement heard through the stethoscope, indicates obstruction of the airway [15].

Fig. 8.3 The
laryngospasm notch

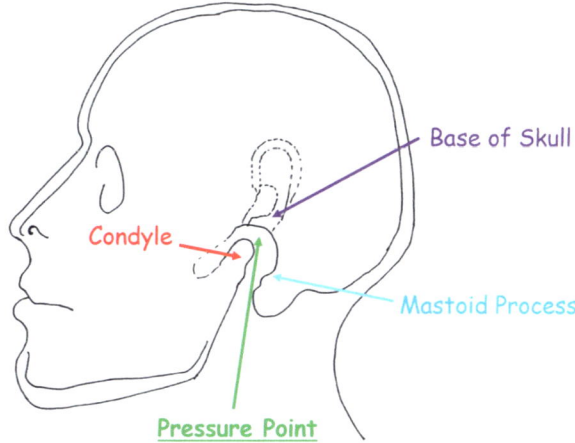

Hypoventilation or respiratory depression is characterized by a shallow depth and rate of chest and abdominal movements, with decreased/no airway movement heard through the stethoscope.

In the two scenarios described above, it should be noted that a pediatric stethoscope is mandatory. Although Basic Life Support (BLS) courses advocate a "look-listen-feel" to assess adequacy of breathing, it is primarily for the lay person or an "outside the clinical area" scenario. The clinician practicing moderate sedation in a child should use a pediatric stethoscope for the same purpose.

Either scenario indicates that exchange of air is not happening. In this situation, the presence of a carotid pulse is quickly confirmed by sliding a couple of fingers from the thyroid cartilage into the groove just before the sternocleidomastoid muscle. The detection of a good pulse confirms that the child is not in cardiac arrest.

Then, in addition to the basic measures described above, repeated deep digital pressure into the "laryngospasm notch" pushing the mandible medially and anteriorly may bring the child to lighter levels of sedation and stimulate spontaneous ventilation [15]. The laryngospasm notch is bounded "anteriorly by the ascending mandibular ramus adjacent to the condyle, posteriorly by the mastoid process, and superiorly by the base of the skull" (Fig. 8.3). Assisted positive pressure ventilation can also be used at this stage as described below.

8.4.4   Assisted Positive Pressure Ventilation

An apparatus to provide positive pressure ventilation (PPV) that includes a 100% oxygen source and a bag valve mask (BVM) device is the most important emergency equipment required for sedation-related emergencies in the dental office. The AAPD recommends the presence of a support personnel, in addition to the practitioner, for moderate sedation. This will help a great deal during emergencies because two rescuers will provide more effective ventilation using the BVM

Fig. 8.4 The E-C clamp
technique

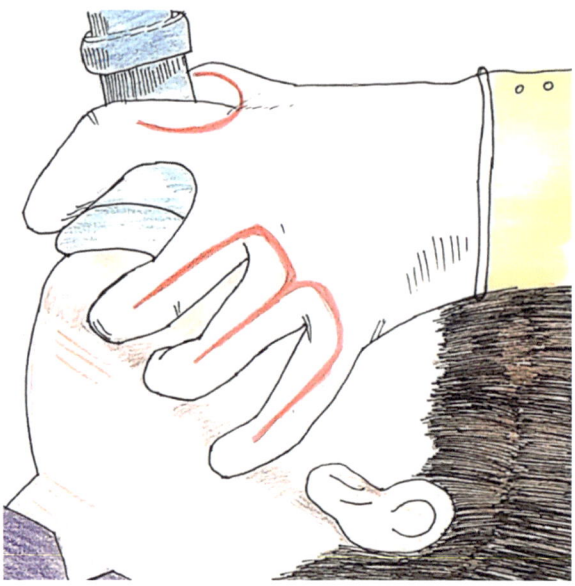

compared to a single rescuer. The practitioner opens the airway with a chin lift and
will establish a tight seal of the mask over the face of the child. The bridge of the
nose is used as a guide for the correct positioning of the mask. The E-C clamp
technique is utilized to hold the mask over the face. The thumb and index finger of
both the hands are used to make a "C" pressing the mask tightly against the face.
The remaining three fingers of each hand make an "E" to lift the angles of the jaw
to open the airway (Fig. 8.4).

The support personnel squeezes the bag completely to give the breaths. For a
child, the rate should be 12–20 breaths/minute. Assisted ventilation with PPV is
confirmed to be effective only if it causes a visible chest rise and audible sounds are
heard through the stethoscope. PPV is continued till the child returns to lighter levels of sedation and spontaneous ventilation.

8.4.5   The Oropharyngeal Airway

If the assisted ventilation is proving ineffective in the unresponsive child (*NO visible chest rise, and audible sounds through the stethoscope*), insertion of an "*oropharyngeal airway*" (OPA) should be considered (Fig. 8.5).

The absence of a gag reflex in the deeply sedated condition will allow insertion
of an OPA. The OPA will supplement the PPV by keeping the tongue away. The
OPA is available in various sizes. The right size of the OPA is selected by placing
one end at the angle of the mouth. The right-sized OPA extends till the angle of the
mandible or slightly beyond (Fig. 8.6).

Fig. 8.5 Oropharyngeal airway

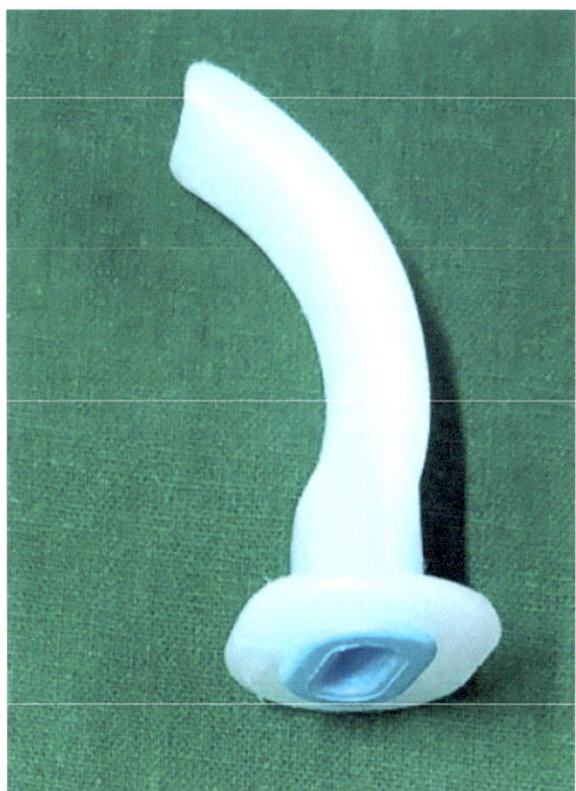

Fig. 8.6 Size selection of the OPA

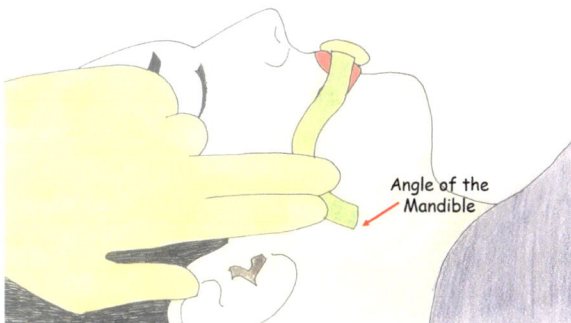

The assisted ventilation *(with visible chest rise, and audible sounds through the stethoscope)* with the BVM and OPA is continued till consciousness *(coughing and gagging, which indicates that the OPA has to be removed)* and spontaneous ventilation returns. If the "single drug-single dose" rule was followed at prescribed midazolam doses, the clinician can self-assure that the short alpha half-life *(clinical*

duration of action) of midazolam will eventually decrease the concentration and bioavailability of the drug in the plasma, thereby ensuring the child's return of consciousness and spontaneous ventilation.

8.4.6   The Use of a Laryngeal Mask Airway

If assisted ventilation proves inadequate in spite of the above measures (*no visible chest rise, and audible sounds*), then emergency medical services (EMS) should be activated. The airway obstruction is very likely below the level of the tongue here. It could be a laryngospasm or bronchospasm (due to possible aspiration of vomitus). At this stage, the insertion of supraglottic airways like the laryngeal mask airway is required as an advanced airway adjunct (Fig. 8.7).

This advanced airway connected to the PPV apparatus provides a direct pathway for the oxygen into the glottis till the EMS arrives. It will also prevent gastric inflation and resultant vomiting and aspiration that can happen because of the ineffective but overzealous PPV. The supraglottic airways are easy to insert. For videos on the method of insertion of an OPA or an LMA, the reader is referred to several excellent resources available on the web [17, 18]. The size selection for the LMA is as follows (Fig. 8.8):

Although endotracheal intubation would have been ideal at this stage, it is a skill set requiring the administration of a depolarizing muscle relaxant like succinylcholine along with extensive clinical training and is not recommended for moderate sedation practitioners.

Fig. 8.7 Laryngeal mask airway

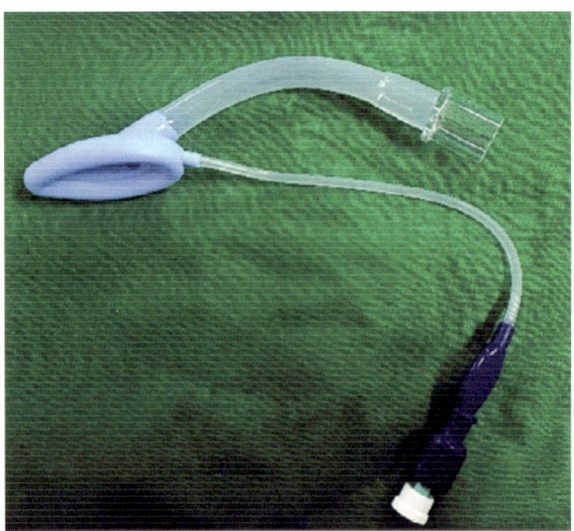

Size of the LMA	1	1.5	2	2.5	3	4	5
Weight of the patient	< 5 Kgs	5-10 Kgs	10-20 Kgs	20-30 Kgs	30 Kgs Young Adult	Adult	Large Adult
Volume of air needed to inflate the cuff (Written also on the LMA)	4 ml	7 ml	10 ml	14 ml	20 ml	30 ml	40 ml

Fig. 8.8 Size selection of LMA

8.4.7 The Administration of Flumazenil

If respiratory depression secondary to midazolam overdosage is suspected, the administration of the reversal agent, flumazenil, intramuscularly can be considered at this stage. It is available as 0.1 mg/mL in 5 mL vials. It is approved for intravenous administration only, at 0.01 mg/kg to a maximum dose of 0.2 mg/dose as the initial dose, to be repeated if necessary. But for an emergency scenario, a higher intramuscular dose has also been suggested at 1 mg (two 5 mL vials of 0.1 mg/mL) [15].

Intranasal administration of flumazenil through a mucosal atomization device (MAD) is another alternative [19]. The dosage recommended is 0.04 mg/kg [20]. A dose of 0.1 mg (1 mL in each of the nares) is also reported to be effective in most children [19].

8.4.8 The Administration of Adrenaline

In a worst-case scenario (*very unlikely in moderate sedation, if the ground rules have been followed except in a rare outlier/hyper-responder*), with the assisted ventilation proving ineffective (*no visible chest rise and audible breath sounds*), the saturation continuing to fall, and the monitors displaying bradycardia, it has to be accepted that the airway emergency has now deteriorated to a cardiac emergency, impending arrest. Adrenaline at 0.01 mg/kg body weight to a maximum dose of 0.3 mg can be administered intramuscularly to increase the heart rate and manage the possible bronchospasm. PPV efforts should continue till the EMS arrives or till consciousness and spontaneous ventilation returns. This is because the primary problem of lack of oxygen if not addressed will lead to severe neurologic morbidity.

8.4.9 The Initiation of Cardiac Compressions

The carotid pulse should be checked every couple of minutes. If a carotid pulse cannot be detected for 10 s, then a cardiac arrest is assumed, and cardiac compressions are to be initiated at 100 compressions per minute. The clinician places the heel of one hand between the nipples with the other hand on top. The compressions should depress the chest to one half its depth and allow complete recoil. The compression ventilation ratio is 15:2 considering a trained assistant is present. If an advanced airway like an LMA is already inserted, then the chest compressions should not be interrupted. The support personnel should give 1 breath simultaneously with the compressions every 6–8 seconds. Five cycles are performed. This is followed by turning on the automated external defibrillator (AED) and following the voice commands. This sequence of compressions, breaths, and AED is continued till the EMS arrives. The reader is referred to a standard Basic Life Support course for further details [21].

8.4.10 Management of Intraoperative Vomiting

The other possible emergency related to sedation that can occur in a dental practice is intraoperative vomiting. This may occur secondary to the NPO rule being violated. When intraoperative vomiting is encountered, an important action is to clear the airway and prevent aspiration. This is made possible by immediately rolling the child to the side, head down, and suctioning the mouth and the pharynx. The Yankauer/tonsillar suctioning tip helps this cause a great deal. It is connected to a high-speed evacuation. It has a widen lumen, made of hard plastic, and is precurved to match the mouth-hypopharynx curvature. It does not get easily clogged and is ideally suited for evacuation of vomitus and debris from the hypopharynx, providing a clear pathway for oxygen to reach the lungs.

8.4.11 List of Emergency Drugs and Equipments

Along with procuring and maintaining the emergency drugs and equipments, the clinician should also learn the skills required to use them. The American Heart Association-affiliated Basic Life Support (BLS) courses, Advanced Cardiac Life Support (ACLS) courses, and Pediatric Advanced Life Support (PALS) aid the clinician develop these skills.

Based on management of the complications described above, here is a list of emergency drugs and equipments including monitoring devices recommended by the authors, for a practice catering to moderate sedation with midazolam in children:

- Shoulder roll
- Bag valve mask device
- Adequate-sized oxygen cylinder and masks
- Oropharyngeal airways
- Laryngeal mask airway
- Flumazenil 5 mL vials, 0.1 mg/mL (2 nos.)
- Adrenaline 1:1000 (1 mg/mL)
- Disposable syringe with a 22 G, 1 inch needle
- Pulse oximeter

- Stethoscope
- Digital sphygmomanometer
- Capnograph (desirable).
- Automated external defibrillator
- Yankauer suction tip

This list is suitable primarily for sedation-related emergencies. Syncope, allergic reactions, asthma, local anesthetic overdoses, foreign body obstructions, and other emergencies may also occur in a pediatric dental setting, which will require additional drugs and equipment. For a more comprehensive reading on the subject of emergencies, drugs, and equipments in the dental clinic, the reader is referred to other excellent, well-established resources on the subject [22].

Clinically Relevant Points
1. Respecting the ground rules for sedation will aid the clinician a long way in forestalling emergencies.
2. A pre-operative assessment helps the clinician classify the child under an ASA category, thereby alerting her/him to the systemic status of a child.
3. The updated NPO guidelines by the European Society for Paediatric Anesthesiology (ESPA) endorsed by the Society for Paediatric Anesthesia of Australia and New Zealand encourage drinking clear fluids till 1 h prior to surgery in elective surgery unless specific contraindications exist.
4. "Single drug-single dose" of a sedative implies that a single drug should be used to obtain minimal/moderate sedation with a single dose.
5. Deep sedation and general anesthesia are a continuum, and the terminology or definitions are only academic.
6. Ideally, the airway should be secured with endotracheal intubation for long dental operatory procedures under general anesthesia. Deep sedation (light planes of general anesthesia) with an open airway should be reserved only for very short dental procedures with judicious use of water and careful placement of a rubber dam.
7. Moderate sedation is essentially a "conscious" technique. The child remains conscious throughout the sedation episode. A brief closure of eyes or sleep should be easily interrupted with light tactile stimulation like a tap on the shoulder.
8. The purpose of monitoring is to provide the clinician with a warning or an alert when there is a change in the recommended physiological parameters in a sedated child.
9. The recovery and discharge protocols rival in importance to all the pre-operative and intraoperative protocols recommended for sedation.
10. The two common respiratory complications of sedation are the obstruction of the airway secondary to loss of the muscle tone and hypoventilation (respiratory depression) secondary to drug overdose, due to loss of the central respiratory drive.

11. The basic management of desaturation in a deeply sedated child involves placing a shoulder roll to raise the torso, suctioning the airway, and a head tilt-chin lift, along with supplemental 100% oxygen delivered via a face mask.

12. The clinician practicing moderate sedation in children should always have a pediatric stethoscope to evaluate the adequacy of breathing.

13. An apparatus to provide positive pressure ventilation (PPV) that includes a 100% oxygen source and a bag valve mask (BVM) device is the most important emergency equipment required for sedation-related emergencies in the dental office.

14. In an emergency scenario, a higher intramuscular dose for flumazenil can be administered intramuscularly at 1 mg (two 5 mL vials of 0.1 mg/mL). Intranasal administration of flumazenil through a mucosal atomizer device (MAD) is another alternative. The dosage recommended is 0.04 mg/kg. A dose of 0.1 mg (1 mL in each of the nares) is also reported to be effective in most children.

15. When intraoperative vomiting is encountered, an important action is to clear the airway. This is made possible by immediately rolling the child to the side, head down, and suctioning the mouth and the pharynx.

References

1. Malamed SF. Prevention. In: Medical emergencies in the dental office. 7th ed. St. Louis, MO: Elsevier; 2015. p. 15–61.
2. Coté CJ, Wilson S. Guidelines for monitoring and management of pediatric patients before, during, and after sedation for diagnostic and therapeutic procedures. Pediatr Dent. 2019;41(4):259–60.
3. Milnes AR, Wilson S. Preoperative assessment and review of systems. In: Wilson S, editor. Oral sedation for dental procedures in children. Berlin: Springer; 2015. p. 25–37.
4. Toms AS, Rai E. Operative fasting guidelines and postoperative feeding in paediatric anaesthesia-current concepts. Indian J Anaesth. 2019;63(9):707–12. https://doi.org/10.4103/ija.IJA_484_19.
5. Korkusuz M, Basaran B, Et T, Bilge A, Yarimoglu R, Osmanoglu UO. Gastric emptying times of obese and non-obese school-aged children after preoperative clear fluid intake: a prospective observational study. Paediatr Anaesth. 2023;33:539. https://doi.org/10.1111/pan.14658.
6. The effect of oral fluid administration 1 hour before surgery on preoperative anxiety and gastric volume in pediatrics. ClinicalTrials.gov identifier: NCT05592964. Updated October 10, 2022. Accessed 30 June 2023. https://clinicaltrials.gov/study/NCT05592964
7. Dalal KS, Rajwade D, Suchak R. "Nil per oral after midnight": is it necessary for clear fluids? Indian J Anaesth. 2010;54(5):445–7. https://doi.org/10.4103/0019-5049.71044.
8. Wilson S. Protocol. In: Wilson S, editor. Oral sedation for dental procedures in children. Berlin: Springer; 2015. p. 113–39.
9. Zanette G, Favero L, Manani G, Facco E. Intranasal flumazenil and naloxone to reverse oversedation in a child undergoing dental restorations: comment. Paediatr Anaesth. 2010;20(1):109. https://doi.org/10.1111/j.1460-9592.2009.03194.

10. Sivaramakrishnan G, Sridharan K. Nitrous oxide and midazolam sedation: a systematic review and meta-analysis. Anesth Prog. 2017;64(2):59–65. https://doi.org/10.2344/anpr-63-03-06.
11. Al-Zahrani AM, Wyne AH, Sheta SA. Comparison of oral midazolam with a combination of oral midazolam and nitrous oxide-oxygen inhalation in the effectiveness of dental sedation for young children. J Indian Soc Pedod Prev Dent. 2009;27(1):9–16. https://doi.org/10.4103/0970-4388.50810.
12. Malamed SF. Oral sedation. In: Sedation: a guide to patient management. 6th ed. St. Louis, MO: Elsevier; 2018. p. 95–119.
13. Malamed SF. Fundamentals of general anesthesia. In: Sedation: a guide to patient management. 6th ed. St. Louis, MO: Elsevier; 2018. p. 407–15.
14. Reed KL, Jo AO. Working with a dentist anesthesiologist. In: Wright GZ, Kupietzky A, editors. Behavior management in dentistry for children. 2nd ed. Wiley Blackwell. p. 177–84.
15. Ganzberg SI. Emergency management. In: Wilson S, editor. Oral sedation for dental procedures in children. Berlin: Springer; 2015.p. p. 195–209.
16. American Academy of Pediatric Dentistry. Behavior guidance for the pediatric dental patient. The reference manual of pediatric dentistry. Chicago, IL: American Academy of Pediatric Dentistry; 2020. p. 292–310.
17. Staffs Paramedics. Oropharyngeal airway insertion. In: YouTube[IN.] Jan 6 2017. https://www.youtube.com/watch?v=Hzc_T4QBp4E. Accessed 6 June 2022.
18. Merck Manuals. How to insert a laryngeal mask airway. In: YouTube[IN] April 9, 2018. https://www.youtube.com/watch?v=NVD18kBjMyQ. Accessed 22 June 2022.
19. Zanette G, Favero L, Manani G, Facco E. Intranasal flumazenil and naloxone to reverse over-sedation in a child undergoing dental restorations: comment. Paediatr Anaesth. 2010;20(1):109. https://doi.org/10.1111/j.1460-9592.2009.03194.x. Epub 2009 Nov 18.
20. Scheepers LD, Montgomery CJ, Kinahan AM, Dunn GS, Bourne RA, McCormack JP. Plasma concentration of flumazenil following intranasal administration in children. Can J Anaesth. 2000;47(2):120–4. https://doi.org/10.1007/BF03018846.
21. Basic Life Support. In: American Heart Association. CPR and first aid emergency cardiovascular care. https://cpr.heart.org/en/cpr-courses-and-kits/healthcare-professional/basic-life-support-bls-training. Accessed 7 July 2023.
22. Malamed SF. Preparation. In: Medical emergencies in the dental office. 7th ed. St. Louis, MO: Elsevier; 2015. p. 62–112.

Documentation

9

9.1 Overview

This chapter explains the documentation required for midazolam sedation in detail. This will include the documentation for drug procurement from the pharmacy along with pre-operative, intraoperative, and post-operative documentation. Detailed annexures with samples for all the above documentation have been provided at the end of the chapter. The reader can modify them to suit her/his practice.

9.2 Background and Objective

Documentation helps reconstruction of events occurring through the sedation procedure. In addition to providing a legal safety net, it also helps the clinician review the case for areas of improvement. The professionalism observed towards meticulous documentation also enhances parent's confidence in the practice. The chapter aims to help the reader understand the documentation associated with midazolam sedation, which is broadly divided into four categories. It begins with the procurement of the drug from the pharmacy. Pre-operative, intraoperative, and post-operative documentation comprise the other three categories. Each section and subsection of the documentation should be numbered and should follow a fixed sequence as depicted below.

9.3 Drug Procurement

Midazolam is listed as a Schedule H drug. According to the Drugs and Cosmetic Rules, 1945, Government of India, Schedule H drugs are a class of prescription drugs that cannot be purchased over the counter [1, 2]. They can be sold by a retailer only against the prescription of a registered medical practitioner and the

© The Author(s), under exclusive license to Springer Nature Switzerland AG 2024
A. Rao, S. Tiwari, *Midazolam in Pediatric Dentistry*,
https://doi.org/10.1007/978-3-031-45147-8_9

maintenance of a documentation trail. The retailer also cannot dispense the prescription more than once, and only the amount prescribed should be dispensed. The prescription should contain the details of the patient, registration details of the doctor along with the address of the practice, signature of the doctor, and date of prescription. The quantity of the drug to be dispensed for the particular patient should be specified. Schedule H drugs cannot be bought and stored in bulk in the practice unless licenses for storage are obtained.

The doctor should maintain a copy of the prescription and account for its use on the patient in the intraoperative documentation.

9.4　Pre-operative Documentation

This includes:

1. Pre-operative assessment records
2. Informed consent
3. Pre-operative parent instructions

9.4.1　Pre-operative Assessment Records

The objective of a pre-operative assessment is to evaluate the systemic status of the child and to categorize her/him in the "American Society of Anesthesiologists" (*ASA*) classification. Only ASA I and ASA II children should be taken up for sedation in the dental OPD [3]. The seven steps to arrive at an ASA category for the child are as follows:

1. A structured medical history
2. Pre-operative vital signs
3. Body mass index (BMI)-for-age percentiles
4. Tonsil size and extraoral anatomic abnormalities
5. Mallampati classification for the child
6. History of upper respiratory tract infection (URTI)
7. Auscultation of the lungs and heart

The reader is referred to Chap. 3 for a detailed explanation of the above steps. Please refer to **Annexure 1** for a sample form of the pre-operative assessment document.

9.4.2　Informed Consent

Informed consent is not just a legal necessity. It is also the moral responsibility of the clinician to educate the parent about the benefits, risks, and alternatives to the proposed intervention. The informed consent should also mention the possible use of protective stabilization. A sample of the informed consent document is given as **Annexure 2**.

9.4.3   Pre-operative Parent Instructions

A set of written pre-operative instructions will help reinforce the verbal instructions given by the clinician to the parent, regarding the treatment under sedation. It is very important especially to reinforce the "nil per oral" (*NPO*) concept and the importance of a healthy upper respiratory tract. The reader is referred to Chap. 8 for a detailed explanation of NPO.

Chapter 3 will provide details on the effect of upper respiratory tract infection on sedation. Written pre-operative instructions will also help parents understand their important role for the overall success of the sedation appointment. Please find a sample of the pre-operative instructions in **Annexure 3**.

9.5   Intraoperative Documentation

This will include four subsections:

(a) Sedation checklist
(b) Drug dosage calculation of midazolam
(c) Time-based sedation record
(d) Intraoperative clinical notes

The purpose of the sedation checklist is to preclude any unexpected problems interfering with the sedation appointment. The status and functioning of the monitors and the emergency equipment including the oxygen apparatus, the suction apparatus, and the dental chair in general should be confirmed and recorded the day before the sedation appointment.

After the patient reaches the office will record any change in the medical history or recent history of upper respiratory tract infections since the last visit. It will also confirm the NPO status of the child and confirm if the wash room pre-operative instructions have been followed and the presence of two accompanying adults.

The dosage for midazolam is calculated according to the weight of the child. The number of ampules used or any ampule wasted is also recorded here.

The time-based record is divided into 15-minutes intervals. All the drugs administered and the vital signs recorded are written in the time-based chart. The sedation level (*University of Michigan Sedation Scale*) [4] and the behavior/responsiveness [5] to treatment are also recorded in the time-based chart. The reader is referred to Chap. 7, Sect. 7.8, for details of the sedation and the behavior scale.

The section ends with "Clinical Notes," which will summarize the entire intraoperative procedure including the time when the procedure started and ended, any special episodes like the child spitting out part of the drug, or any other complications encountered during the procedure.

A sample of the intraoperative documentation is given in **Annexure 4**.

9.6   Post-operative Documentation

This will include:

(a) Discharge criteria
(b) Post-operative parent instructions and discharge summary

9.6.1   Discharge Criteria

Managing the post-operative phase of the sedation is as important as the pre-operative and intraoperative parts. It has major child safety implications. A checklist against which the child will be discharged to a responsible adult, guards against any laxity that may set in post a taxing sedation appointment. Please find in **Annexure 5** a sample of the document check listing the discharge criteria.

9.6.2   Post-operative Parent Instructions and Discharge Summary

Written post-operative parent instructions should be reviewed with the parents before discharge [6]. It will help parents be more proactive and alert and also prevent small problems from becoming real emergencies.

The discharge summary sums up the entire case starting pre-operatively and ending with the discharge of the child. It is given to the caregiver as a healthcare record, which will accompany the child to any subsequent consultations by other health professionals. **Annexure 6** is a sample of the post-operative parent instructions and the discharge summary.

Clinically Relevant Points
1. Midazolam is listed as a Schedule H drug. It can be sold by a retailer only against the prescription of a registered medical practitioner.
2. Schedule H drugs cannot be bought and stored in bulk in the practice unless licenses for storage are obtained.
3. Pre-operative documentation includes pre-operative assessment records, informed consent, and pre-operative parent instructions.
4. Intraoperative documentation includes a sedation checklist, drug dosage calculation of midazolam, time-based sedation record, and intraoperative clinical notes.
5. Post-operative documentation will include discharge criteria and post-operative parent instructions and discharge summary.

Annexure 1: Pre-operative Assessment

Medical Questionnaire

Dear Parent,

Dental treatment plans have to be made based on the child's medical history. So, in order to make an ideal and safe dental treatment plan for your child, please fill out the following medical history questionnaire to the best of your knowledge.

Date:

Child's Name: Date of Birth:

Sex: Male/Female   Frankl Behaviour Rating:
                                                    (to be filled by the clinician)

1. Name of the child's physician with phone number……………………………………………………
2. Any recent visit to the child's physician…………………Yes/No
3. Is the child on any regular medication or any recent medications?………………………Yes/No
4. Has the child been hospitalized in the past for any reason?………………………………Yes/No
5. Any abnormal bleeding associated with previous surgery or falls during play or during any other accident…………………………………………………… …………………………………………………………….Yes/No
6. Any recent X-rays, lab tests, or other investigations…………………………………………………Yes/No
7. Is the child allergic to any drug, food, or any other substance?…………………………Yes/No
8. Was the child's delivery premature?………………………………………………………Yes/No
9. Does the child snore at night?……………………………………………………………… …………Yes/No
10. Is the child exposed to passive smoking?…………………………………………………………………..Yes/no
11. Does the child have (or had) a diagnosed medical health problem? …………………………Yes/No
12. If yes, can you please indicate it from the list below?

Heart disease	Allergy to food/medicine/others	Asthma/breathing problems	Fainting spells
Hepatitis/jaundice/liver disease	Childhood diabetes	Frequent painful/swollen joints	Kidney problems
Tuberculosis	Thyroid problems	AIDS/HIV	Psychiatric counseling
Anemia	Physical/developmental disability	Seizures/epilepsy	Any other problem the dentist should know

13. Any previous dental visits..
....Yes/No

14. If yes, any serious problem with previous dental treatments
To the best of my knowledge, all the preceding answers are true and correct. In case of any change, I will inform the doctor without fail.

Parent signature and date:

Doctor's signature and date:

Pre-operative Vital Signs

Pulse rate, rhythm, quality:
   Respiratory rate:
   Oxygen saturation:
   Blood pressure:

Examination of the Tonsil Size

Normal/enlarged/kissing tonsils:

The Mallampati Score

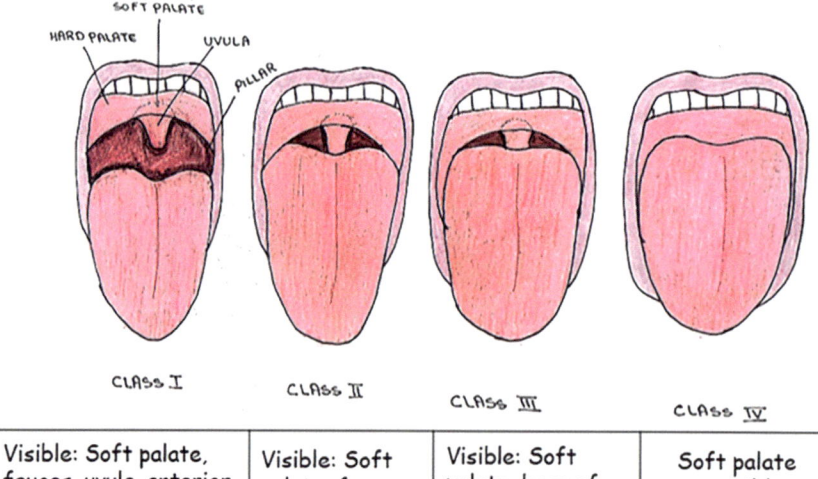

Visible: Soft palate, fauces, uvula, anterior and posterior pillars	Visible: Soft palate, fauces, uvula	Visible: Soft palate, base of uvula	Soft palate not visible

History of Active Upper Respiratory Tract Infection (URTI) in the Last 4 Weeks

Coughing, active nasal discharge, wheezing/crackles, history of asthma, recent history of antibiotics for a URTI

BMI-for-Age Percentiles to Check for Obesity

Height:
Weight:
BMI-for-age percentiles: Normal/overweight/underweight

Auscultation of the Lungs and Heart

Accessory heart sounds: Yes/No
Abnormal breath sounds: Yes/No

ASA Score (Based on Information Above)

ASA I/ASA II/ASA III/ASA IV
Signature of the doctor with date:

Annexure 2: Informed Consent Form for Midazolam Sedation

Patient Name/Age/Gender/Weight: Date:

Recommended Treatment

Dental treatment under midazolam sedation
Route of midazolam administration: _____

Treatment Alternatives

Alternative methods of treatment are deferring the treatment temporarily with medications or completing the treatment under general anesthesia.

Risks and Complications

I understand that there are risks and complications associated with the administration of midazolam.

These potential risks and complications include, but are not limited to, the following:

1. Vomiting and aspiration if feeding instructions are not followed
2. Loss of consciousness
3. Allergic reaction
4. Failure to achieve any sedation
5. Prolonged sluggishness in motion and/or speech
6. Abnormal/shallow breathing
7. Hiccups

Any of these complications may require emergency medical attention and/or hospitalization.

I, the undersigned, acknowledge that Dr. _____ has explained to me that my child has to undergo dental treatment under midazolam sedation.

I have been explained that protective stabilization in the form of papoose board, mouth props, or gentle restraint of the child's head or extremities may be necessary during the sedation appointment, to prevent sudden movements by the child.

I have been explained that nitrous oxide-oxygen may be used to further supplement the midazolam sedation and provide analgesia (pain relief).

I have been explained the need for the nature of the procedure and its possible side effects, risks, benefits, alternatives, and complications. I have understood the same and give my free and informed consent for the same to be performed.

I am also aware that I should not give anything to eat or drink to my child and see that she/he does not eat or drink on her/his own _____ hours before the procedure as it can cause serious complications during the procedure.

I also acknowledge strongly that I have disclosed all the medical problems, if any, regarding my child to the above said doctor.

I certify and acknowledge that I have read and understood the contents of this form. It has been read and explained to me in a language understood by me.

Name/age/gender/signature of person giving the above stated consent:

Relation with the patient:

Date and time:

Name and signature of doctor taking the consent:

Doctor's additional remarks:

Annexure 3: Pre-operative Parent Instructions

Name of the patient:

Date:

As discussed in the consultation appointment, your child requires dental treatment to be completed under midazolam sedation.

Midazolam is expected to decrease the child's anxiety. It will calm and relax the child. It may cause moderate sedation (drowsiness) and ideally some amnesia (child will not remember what transpired during the dental procedure). The child is expected to remain interactive and awake during the dental procedure.

Kindly follow the instructions below:

- The child should be well rested before the sedation appointment. A restless child could get cranky under the effect of midazolam.
- Please bring another adult to the sedation appointment who would be able to drive while you can take care of the child in the journey back home.
- The child can bring her/his favorite toy or blanket to the appointment.
- Child should be dressed in a comfortable and loose-fitting clothing on the day of the sedation appointment.
- Please call the dental office if the child develops cold, flu, fever, or congestion 24 hours before the appointment.
- Please follow the feeding instructions strictly. Clear fluids should be avoided within 2 hours of the sedative administration, breast milk within 4 hours, light meals including non-human milk within 6 hours, and fatty meals within 8 hours. Please call the clinic in case of doubt. An empty stomach is necessary to prevent vomiting during the dental treatment.
- The child should use the washroom at home before coming to the dental office for the sedation appointment. The child can wear a diaper if toilet training is not fully established.

Signature of the doctor:

Annexure 4: Intraoperative Documentation

Name of the patient:
   Date:

Sedation Appointment Checklist

- Functioning of the pulse oximeter.
- Functioning of the oxygen cylinder.
- Functioning of the suction apparatus.
- Functioning of the dental chair.
- Check emergency equipments list.
- Any change in the medical history.
- Any history of upper respiratory tract infections since the last visit.
- NPO (nil per oral) status.
- Compliance with washroom instructions.
- Presence of two adults.

Midazolam Dosage Calculation (Example Below)

Route: Oral
   Child weight: 16 kg
   Dosage: at 0.5 mg/kg body weight of midazolam = 8 mg of midazolam
   Number of 5 mg/mL midazolam ampules required: 2 (1.6 mL)
   Remarks:

Time-Based Record

	Baseline (9.00 AM)	9.15	9.30	9.45	10.00	10.15	10.30	10.45	11.00	11.15	11.45
Midazolam (mg)											
N_2O/O_2 %											
Local anesthetic (mg)											
Sedation level											
Behavior											
SpO_2											
Respiratory rate/minute											
Quality of breath sounds (normal = N)											
Heart rate											
Temperature											
Blood pressure											

Clinical Notes

Signature of the doctor:

Annexure 5: Discharge Criteria

Name of the patient:
    Date:

- The child is responding to her/his name (if age appropriate).
- The child is sitting up unaided (if age appropriate) without dizziness.
- No signs of disorientation.
- Vital signs close to baseline.
  - SpO_2
  - Respiratory rate
  - Quality of breath sounds
  - Heart rate
  - Blood pressure
  - Temperature
- The child has stayed awake for 20 min (University of Michigan Sedation Scale, value 0) in a quiet environment.
- Post-operative instructions reviewed with the caregiver.
- Child discharged to two adults each responsible for driving the vehicle and observing the child, respectively.

Annexure 6: Post-operative Parent Instructions and Discharge Summary

Name of the patient:
    Date:

Post-operative Parent Instructions
- Medications to be given to the child as prescribed.
- The soft tissues will be numb (lips, cheeks, tongue) because of the local anesthetic injection for another couple of hours. Please observe the child against lip biting or any other soft tissue trauma.
- On the way home, one adult will be in charge of driving the vehicle, and the other will be monitoring the child. Should the child wish to sleep on the way home, the airway should be kept open and chin off the chest with a head tilt.
- Once home, the child should be started initially on clear fluids. If the child accepts it well, soft foods can be started in small portions. Avoid large portions and fatty foods. The child should be well hydrated, especially for the next 24 hours.

- The child could sleep more in the next 24-hours period. During sleep, the child should be on her/his side and not in the supine position. Pillows can be placed on the back and the abdomen to stabilize the child in this position. *Do not place a pillow near the child's face.*
- Parents should periodically monitor the sleeping child in general and specifically for any episodes of vomiting.
- When awake, the child should not be playing alone and should always be under close adult supervision for the next 24 hours. The child may be unsteady or dizzy, and activities like bicycle riding or climbing stairs is a strict no-no. The child could also be irritable for 24 hours.

Discharge Summary
Date of first consultation:
Chief complaint:
Diagnosis:
Treatment plan:
Reason for treatment under midazolam sedation:
Date of the sedation appointment:
Dosage of midazolam administered with route:
Any complications:
Medications at discharge:
Clinical notes:

Signature of the doctor with date:

References

1. Pharma Franchise Help. Schedule H: Prescription of drugs. https://pharmafranchisehelp.com/drug-cosmetic-act-rules-schedule-h-list-prescription-drugs/. Accessed 7 July 2022
2. Med India. Drugs and cosmetic rules—schedule H and Schedule H 1 drugs. October 17, 2019. https://www.medindia.net/patientinfo/drugs-and-cosmetics-rules-schedule-h-schedule-h1-drugs.htm. Accessed 7 July 2022
3. Milnes AR, Wilson S. Preoperative assessment and review of systems. In: Wilson S, editor. Oral sedation for dental procedures in children. Berlin: Springer; 2015. p. 25–37.
4. Malviya S, Voepel-Lewis T, Tait AR, Merkel S, Tremper K, Naughton N. Depth of sedation in children undergoing computed tomography: validity and reliability of the University of Michigan Sedation Scale (UMSS). Br J Anaesth. 2002;88(2):241–5.
5. AAPD. Sedation Record. https://www.aapd.org/globalassets/media/policies_guidelines/r_sedationrecord.pdf. Accessed 23 April 2022
6. Wilson S. Protocol. In: Wilson S, editor. Oral sedation for dental procedures in children. Berlin: Springer; 2015. p. 113–39.